European School of Oncology

Monographs

Series Editor: U. Veronesi

The European School of Oncology
gratefully acknowledges sponsorship
for the Task Force received from

Roche

Springer

Berlin
Heidelberg
New York
Barcelona
Budapest
Hong Kong
London
Milan
Paris
Tokyo

L. Degos D.R. Parkinson (Eds.)

Retinoids in Oncology

With 26 Figures and 10 Tables

Springer

Professor Laurent Degos

Institut Universitaire d'Hématologie
Hôpital St. Louis
1, Avenue Claude Vellefaux
75010 Paris, France

David R. Parkinson, M.D.

Investigational Drug Branch
Division of Cancer Treatment
National Cancer Institute
6130 Executive Boulevard
Rockville, MD 20892, USA

ISBN-13: 978-3-642-79708-8 e-ISBN-13:978-3-642-79706-4
DOI:10.1007/978-3-642-79706-4

CIP data applied for.

Typesetting: Camera ready by editor
Printing: Druckhaus Beltz, Hemsbach/Bergstraße; Binding: J. Schäffer GmbH & Co. KG, Grünstadt
SPIN: 10132207 19/3133 - 5 4 3 2 1 0 — Printed on acid-free paper

Foreword

The European School of Oncology came into existence to respond to a need for information, education and training in the field of the diagnosis and treatment of cancer. There are two main reasons why such an initiative was considered necessary. Firstly, the teaching of oncology requires a rigorously multidisciplinary approach which is difficult for the Universities to put into practice since their system is mainly disciplinary orientated. Secondly, the rate of technological development that impinges on the diagnosis and treatment of cancer has been so rapid that it is not an easy task for medical faculties to adapt their curricula flexibly.

With its residential courses for organ pathologies and the seminars on new techniques (laser, monoclonal antibodies, imaging techniques etc.) or on the principal therapeutic controversies (conservative or mutilating surgery, primary or adjuvant chemotherapy, radiotherapy alone or integrated), it is the ambition of the European School of Oncology to fill a cultural and scientific gap and, thereby, create a bridge between the University and Industry and between these two and daily medical practice.

One of the more recent initiatives of ESO has been the institution of permanent study groups, also called task forces, where a limited number of leading experts are invited to meet once a year with the aim of defining the state of the art and possibly reaching a consensus on future developments in specific fields of oncology.

The ESO Monograph series was designed with the specific purpose of disseminating the results of these study group meetings, and providing concise and updated reviews of the topic discussed.

It was decided to keep the layout relatively simple, in order to restrict the costs and make the monographs available in the shortest possible time, thus overcoming a common problem in medical literature: that of the material being outdated even before publication.

Umberto Veronesi
Chairman Scientific Committee
European School of Oncology

Contents

Introduction

Laurent Degos [1] and David R. Parkinson [2]

1 Institut Universitaire d'Hématologie, Hôpital St. Louis, 1, Avenue Claude Vellefaux, 75010 Paris, France
2 Investigational Drug Branch, Division of Cancer Treatment, National Cancer Institute, Bethesda, MD 20892, U.S.A.

The retinoids consist of a family of compounds structurally and functionally related to all-*trans*-retinoic acid, the physiologically active metabolite of vitamin A. While the biology of this class of agents has long been of interest to developmental biologists and to those interested in the physiology of vision, it is much more recently that investigators concerned with the prevention and treatment of malignancy have focussed on this class of agents. This recent attention has been fuelled by the rapid increases in our understanding of the normal biology of the retinoids, the appreciation of their powerful influences on gene expression, and the demonstration of their ability in some preclinical settings to interfere with the malignant process.

In this monograph we have attempted to integrate the latest findings from both basic laboratory and clinical research regarding the retinoids. Our purpose has been to summarise under one cover and in a timely manner the spectrum of findings regarding retinoid biology, activity in preclinical model systems, and results from initial therapeutic applications in humans. We have been joined in this project by a knowledgeable and experienced group of individuals who have worked together to produce a summary of this extensive amount of information. The role of natural retinoids in growth and development and the latest information concerning both the structure and function of nuclear retinoid receptors and the mechanisms through which the retinoids influence gene expression are summarised by Zelent. The cell biological consequences of retinoid action on normal, premalignant, and malignant cells are then described by Lotan. The role of retinoids and their receptors in embryogenesis is explained by Morriss-Kay. These three initial chapters represent comprehensive summaries of a huge body of information, and form a basis for understanding the rationales and strategies for the use of retinoids in clinical applications in individuals at risk for malignancy, and in patients with established cancer. The pharmacology of the retinoids, emphasising the differences which have been found among the retinoids used clinically to date, is then summarised by Pastorino, Warrell and Formelli. The need for detailed pharmacological study of each new retinoid is emphasised by the surprising findings with respect to all-*trans* retinoic acid, which differs so remarkably in this respect from its stereoisomer, 13-*cis* retinoic acid. Warrell, Pastorino and Decensi then summarise the acute and chronic toxicities of the retinoids, emphasising the "retinoic acid syndrome" which has been encountered only with the use of all-*trans* retinoic acid in therapy of acute promyelocytic leukaemia (APL), and the ocular toxicities encountered with the use of fenretinide in chemoprevention studies. The effects of all-*trans* RA in APL are then described in a chapter by de Thé, Degos and Warrell which attempts to integrate the clinical effects with progress in the understanding of the molecular and cellular biology of this malignancy. The clinical finding of this therapeutic effect, first described by Professor Huang and his colleagues in China, must rank with some of the most remarkable therapeutic findings in cancer treatment. Beyond its relevance to the treatment of this particular malignancy, the appreciation that the mechanism of the antitumour effects is through induction of differentiation has represented a profound stimulus for studies into differentiation and apoptosis induction as therapeutic strategies in malignancy. The more limited, and less dramatic, therapeutic experiences in other haematological malignancies and premalignant states are then summarised by Parkinson and Warrell. Finally, Pastorino, Parkinson and Chiesa have integrated into one chapter the latest information concerning the use of retinoids in the prevention and therapy of solid tumours. Traditionally these subjects, prevention and therapy, have been separated, both with respect to organisation of meetings and organisation of manuscripts. It increasingly has become clear that both groups of investigators have much to learn from each other, and furthermore, that the conduct of secondary chemoprevention trials is in fact the conduct of adjuvant therapy trials. While clinical and laboratory endpoints for prevention and treatment may differ, and the number of patients in a trial necessary to answer the prevention question be larger than those necessary for the therapeutic goals, the trial design issues, and the populations of patients under therapy are identical. The most efficient path to solving important cancer management questions therefore may lie with increased cooperation between prevention- and treatment-directed clinical researchers.

On behalf of the entire group of authors we would like to express our personal appreciation to the staff of the European School of Oncology for their assistance in this project. We have produced this monograph under an accelerated schedule in order to make available to the reader the latest information concerning retinoids and malignancy. It is our sincere hope that these efforts will prove useful to all those interested in the development and application of new therapies or preventive strategies for cancer.

Molecular Mechanisms of Retinoid Action

Arthur Zelent

Leukaemia Research Fund Centre at the Institute of Cancer Research, Chester Beatty Laboratories, Fulham Road, London SW3 6JB, United Kingdom

Shortly after the discovery of vitamin A (retinol) in 1913 [1], scientists began to realise the extreme importance of this simple fat-soluble molecule in a large number of complex and diverse physiological processes such as vision, reproduction, as well as the development and homeostasis of vertebrates (see ref. [2-9] for reviews). Over the years considerable effort has been devoted to study the cellular metabolism of vitamin A and to characterise its biologically active derivatives (see ref. [10] for review). The term retinoids has been used to encompass a continuously growing family of synthetic and natural compounds which are both structurally and functionally related to vitamin A and its physiologically active metabolites, such as all-*trans*-retinoic acid (RA). By the end of the 1960s the role of retinoids in the visual cycle was well understood [11], however, the molecular mechanism of retinoid action in processes other than vision remained elusive for the next 2 decades. The discovery of a nuclear retinoic acid receptor (RAR) [12,13], which was shown to be a member of the superfamily of steroid/thyroid hormone nuclear receptors [14-16] functioning as ligand-inducible transcription factors, was a breakthrough in understanding how retinoids exert their pleiotropic effects.

Regulation of gene expression at the transcriptional level is an essential component of important cellular and developmental processes such as growth, differentiation and lineage commitment. In this respect, the concerted action of cell-type specific transcription factors, which bind to the DNA elements (response elements) located in the regulatory regions (such as promoters and/or enhancers) of specific genes and either inhibit or stimulate the rate of transcription initiation by DNA polymerase II, is of extreme importance. Nuclear receptors, such as steroid receptors or RARs, are soluble proteins which can bind as dimers to specific DNA-regulatory elements (hormone response elements) and act as cell-type and promoter specific transcription factors. In contrast to other transcription factors, however, their activities can be modulated through binding of the corresponding hydrophobic ligands such as steroid hormones or retinoids. The aim of this chapter is to provide the reader with a comprehensive summary of what has been learned about the molecular components of the retinoid signalling pathway and the mechanisms of their action in physiological processes other than visual perception.

Natural Retinoids and Development

Early work on the effects of vitamin A deficiency in a number of mammalian species implicated it in the control of normal differentiation and proliferation of epithelial cells [3]. This loss of control in a vitamin A deficient animal was reflected in structural and functional abnormalities of various organs and tissues such as the skin, thymus and prostate, as well as the tracheobronchial, urogenital and gastro-intestinal epithelia [3,17]. For example, in the absence of dietary retinol, the secretory and stratified squamous epithelia undergo keratinization (squamous metaplasia) and hyperkeratinization, respectively. Hypervitaminosis A also was found to have deleterious effects on epidermal differentiation causing decreased keratinization and hair loss (see [18] and references therein). It is perhaps not surprising that these early observations led scientists to consider the use of retinoids in cancer therapy (see [19] for review) and treatment of cutaneus disorders of keratinization (for review see [20] and references therein). The action of vitamin A in controlling cellular proliferation and differentiation was not, however, restricted to epithelial cells (see [21,22] for reviews). Avitaminosis A was also associated with a reduction in the number of haemopoietic cells in the bone marrow [3] and anaemia [23]. An important role for retinoids in haemopoiesis was corroborated by studies demonstrating that all-*trans* RA can stimulate the proliferation and maturation of erythroid and myeloid precursor cells *in vitro* [24], and exert beneficial effects on the function of the human immune system (see [25] and references therein). Indeed, recent experimental results [26] have shown that 9-*cis* retinoic acid (9-*cis* RA), a stereoisomer of all-*trans* RA, may play a role in T-cell selection.

Given the observations that avitaminosis or hypervitaminosis A adversely affects most, if not all, cells in adult vertebrate organisms, it was considered very likely that vitamin A and its derivatives would also play an important role during embryogenesis. Early indirect evidence for such a role came from observations of the teratogenic effects of both retinoid deficiency and excess on embryonic development [4,5,27]. Interestingly, the spectrum of malformations produced by these two different conditions were very similar and included primarily skeletal and eye defects, as well as limb, craniofacial, cardiovascular, central nervous system (CNS) and urogenital malformations. The nature of these observed embryonic defects was highly dependent on the stages of maternal exposure [28,29], indicating specific intervals of retinoid sensitivity during the development of various anatomical structures and organ systems. These periods of sensitivity probably reflect developmental windows during which activities of endogenous retinoid are required for proper functioning of normal physiological processes such as programmed cell death (apoptosis) and/or migration of neural crest cells. Indeed, non-physiological levels of retinoid(s) have been associated with abnormal migration of neural crest cells [30] and excessive apoptosis [31,32].

More direct evidence for the role of retinoids in embryogenesis came from studies on avian limb morphogenesis (see [33, 34] and references therein). In 1968 Saunders and Gasseling [35] described a region of mesenchymal cells in the posterior margin of the developing chicken limb bud, named zone of polarising activity (ZPA), that, when transplanted to the anterior margin, would induce mirror image digit duplication. These results led to the suggestion that ZPA was the source of a diffusable morphogen whose concentration gradient across the antero-posterior axis of the limb bud would specify positional values required for proper digit patterning [36]. Possibly influenced by the earlier observations of Niazi and Saxena on the adverse effects of the excess of vitamin A on amphibian tail [37] and limb [38] regeneration, and/or by the nature of all-*trans* RA-induced limb malformations in mammals [29], Tickle and co-workers [39] implanted in the anterior region of the limb bud an anion exchange bead soaked in all-*trans* RA. They discovered that the released all-*trans* RA induced the same pattern of digit duplication as transplanted ZPA, and suggested that all-*trans* RA may indeed be the putative ZPA morphogen. Further support for this hypothesis came in 1987 from Eichele and Thaller [40] who showed that all-*trans* RA can be isolated from chicken limb buds and that its concentration is approximately 2.5-fold higher in the posterior (ZPA-containing) than in the anterior region. Since this time, endogenous retinoids such as all-*trans*-3,4-didehydroretinoic acid and 9-*cis* RA have also been shown to be potent inducers of digit duplication [41,42]. Nevertheless, despite the initial excitement [43] the role of retinoids as morphogens during chicken limb development remains very controversial ([44], see also [34] for review and references therein). In fact, recent results [45,46] suggest that retinoids act not as morphogens but as ZPA inducers, i.e., they simply convert the cells that they come into contact with to ZPA cells and subsequently are not required for polarising activity. This was illustrated by an experiment which showed that when a wedge of tissue next to the all-*trans* RA-releasing bead is cleared from all-*trans* RA and implanted in the anterior margin of another limb bud, it still causes digit duplication. The most recent results have shown that all-*trans* RA can induce expression of a gene called *Sonic hedgehog*, whose product is strongly associated with the polarising activity in the chicken limb bud [47].

Interestingly, *Sonic hedgehog* is a homologue of a *Drosophila* segment polarity gene, *hedgehog*, which may indeed function as a classical morphogen.

Regardless as to whether retinoids act as true morphogens, the results summarised above strongly support the role for these compounds in limb development. Further support for this role comes from studies which have shown that all-*trans* RA can also respecify positional information in the regenerating amphibian limb [48]. As in other systems, the effects of all-*trans* RA on pattern formation in regenerating amphibian limbs are dependent on retinoid concentration, length of treatment and the developmental stage at which retinoid exposure occurs. It is worth pointing out, however, that in contrast to chick limb development, where all-*trans* RA can respecify positional information only in the antero-posterior axis, during limb regeneration in amphibians all-*trans* RA can affect pattern formation along all 3 axes (see [49] for review).

Work carried out initially on *Xenopus laevis* embryos suggests that endogenous retinoids may also have an important role in the formation of the primary embryonic axis [50,51]. Increasing concentrations of exogenous all-*trans* RA applied during early stages of frog embryogenesis were found to progressively transform anterior brain structures into more posterior neural tissues. It is worth noting that this "posteriorising" effect of all-*trans* RA on the antero-posterior body axis of the frog embryo is analogous to its effect on the chicken limb bud development where it also induces essentially an antero-posterior transformation. An all-*trans* RA metabolite, all-*trans*-4-oxo-retinoic acid, which previously was thought to be inactive [33], was recently found to be more potent than all-*trans* RA in modulating this positional specification [52]. Interestingly, this retinoid had lower potency than all-*trans* RA in regulating cellular growth and differentiation, suggesting that various retinoids may affect different physiological processes. Both all-*trans* RA and all-*trans*-4-oxo-retinoic acid were present endogenously in frog embryos [52]. Polarising activities, presumably due to endogenous retinoids such as all-*trans* RA and all-*trans*-3,4-didehydroretinoic acid, have been detected in the Hensen's node and the floor plate isolated from mouse and chick embryos, respectively [53,54], suggesting that these structures may be the sources of retinoids involved in axial specifications.

The effects of retinoids on axial patterning have also been studied in birds and mammals. For example, implantation of all-*trans* RA-soaked anion exchange beads into the anterior side of the antero-posterior axis of gastrulation stage chick embryos caused body axis duplication [55]. Additionally, exposure of early mouse embryos to teratogenic doses of all-*trans* RA caused stage-dependent homeotic transformations of vertebrae [56]. Both posterior and anterior transformations were observed and these were strictly associated with all-*trans* RA treatment at day 7 and 8.5 of development, respectively. Taken together, the data reviewed above are in agreement with earlier observations on the teratogenic effects of retinoids and strongly implicate these compounds as important signalling molecules functioning in vertebrate development.

Retinoids and Control of Gene Expression

The effects of retinoids on pattern formation as well as cellular growth and differentiation have been associated with changes in the levels of expression of specific genes. This has been perhaps best illustrated by the effects of retinoids on the expression of homeobox genes (for review see [57] and references therein). In analogy with their function in *Drosophila*, it is believed that the products of vertebrate class I homeobox-containing (Hox) genes, which encode transcription factors with a characteristic developmentally conserved helix-turn-helix DNA-binding domain (homeodomain), function in specifying positional values within a number of developmental systems [58,59]. Phenotypic changes resulting from either a gain or loss of function mutation in a number of Hox genes are consistent with these beliefs [59-62]. Hox genes are grouped into 4 different clusters (A-D, see [63]) and are expressed during embryonic development in a spatio-temporal manner which reflects their 3' to 5' order in a given cluster, i.e., the more 3' the location of a gene within a cluster, the earlier it is expressed and the more anterior is the boundary of its expression [64]. Amazingly, recent results have shown that in teratocarcinoma cells, the ability of various concentrations of all-*trans* RA to induce the expression of different Hox genes within a given cluster follows the same 3' to 5' polarity, with genes in the more 3' positions being induced by progressively lower concentrations of all-*trans* RA [65]. Furthermore, excess retinoid treatment, which induces antero-posterior transformation of the vertebrae and CNS, as well as digit duplication, alters the pattern of Hox gene expression along the respective antero-posterior axes [66,67]. Therefore, it would appear that retinoids may exert their polarising effects through sequential activation and/or repression of Hox gene expression along the antero-posterior axis. Altering the pattern of Hox gene expression by means other than retinoid treatment (ectopic expression, for example) produces analogous transformations [62]. These results further support the view that the Hox genes are involved in the positional specification and reaffirm the important role of retinoids in pattern formation, perhaps through direct and/or indirect regulation of Hox gene expression.

Another class of molecules with possible morphogenic activities are peptide growth factors (PGFs). Like retinoids, PGFs can induce body axis formation while specifically regulating the expression of various Hox genes [68]. Members of the transforming growth factor ß (TGF-ß) family (activin and bone morphogenic protein 2, for example), and basic fibroblast growth factor and related molecules, have been implicated in the above processes and have been thought to function as concentration-dependent morphogens in amphibian development [69]. Although retinoids and PGFs may act alone to exert their effects, it is likely that a close cooperation between these two distinct classes of signalling molecules exists during development, perhaps at the level of regulation of Hox gene expression. This hypothesis is supported by results showing that all-*trans* RA strongly potentiates the effects of basic fibroblast growth factor on patterning [70] and regulates the mRNA levels of TGF-ßs [71].

Regulation of gene expression by retinoids, Hox gene products and PGFs during development most likely involves complex cross-regulatory interactions between a large number of transcription factors. Examples of such genes are members of the POU [72], PAX [73] and Kruppel-related (Krox-20, Krox-24, mkr genes for example) (see [74] for review) families of transcription factors. Expression of some of these genes, Krox-24 and Oct-3, for example, has been shown to be regulated by retinoids [75,76]. Recently the Krox-20 protein, which is expressed specifically in rhombomers 3 and 5 during hind brain development, has been shown to regulate expression of the HoxB2 gene [77]. Since retinoids can respecify the patterns of expression of HoxB2 and Krox-20 genes in the hind brain and adversely affect its development, it will be most interesting to explore the relationship between the retinoids and the hierarchy of regulatory genes which specify rhombomeric identities.

In addition to the above examples, a whole plethora of genes whose levels of expression are regulated by retinoids have been described [78]. These include transcription factors implicated in protein kinase A and/or C signalling such as AP-2 and NF-κB [79,80], PGF receptors [81], various proteases and metalloproteases [82], which may play roles in tissue remodelling, cell adhesion molecules [83], protooncogenes [84], metabolic enzymes [85,86] and cytoskeletal proteins such as laminins and keratins [87,88]. Clearly not all of these genes are primary targets of retinoid action but may be part of a regulatory cascade involving retinoids, Krox and Hox genes as well as other transcription factors. In this respect, the promoters of some of the above genes, such as the neural cell adhesion molecule, contain Hox regulatory sequences [89]. The effects of retinoids on keratin gene expression reflect the important role that these compounds play in epidermal morphogenesis [90]. It is worth pointing out that, as in embryogenesis, the interactions between the retinoid and PGF signalling pathways (TGF-ßs for example) [91] have been observed during the processes of epidermal differentiation. This suggests that once a certain regulatory network evolves it can be adapted to a number of distinct developmental systems.

Given such a wide range of genes whose expression is affected by retinoids, it is perhaps not surprising that retinoids can also modulate the levels of gene expression of various human and non-human pathogenic viruses. Viruses whose genes have been shown to be regulated directly or indirectly by retinoids include human papillomavirus-18 [92], human immunodeficiency virus [93], cytomegalovirus (CMV) [94], Epstein-Barr virus [95], mouse mammary tumour virus [96] and hepatitis B virus (HBV) [97]. It is worth noting that nearly all of the above viruses have been implicated in tumorigenesis. In this respect, inhibition of human papillomavirus-18 gene expression by retinoids may prove to have therapeutic implications in treatment of cervical carcinomas [92].

It is clear from the above examples that retinoids occupy important positions within a number of gene networks whose functions are important to various cellular and developmental processes. I anticipate that in the near future, the only comprehensive way to illustrate the extent of retinoid action and/or interaction with the above genes and gene networks will be through complex diagrams analogous to the maps worked out decades ago to represent the metabolic pathways and their components.

Retinoid Receptors

In analogy to the steroid hormones [98] the effects of retinoids on cellular growth and differentiation are inseparable from their effects on gene expression. This observation suggested that retinoids may also act through binding to intracellular receptors and encouraged scientists in the field to look for cellular retinoid-binding proteins. This initial effort culminated in 1973 with the discovery by Frank Chytil and co-workers of a cellular retinol-binding protein [99]. Since then a number of other related retinol and retinoic acid binding proteins (CRBPs and CRABPs, respectively) have been purified and their corresponding cDNAs have been cloned (for review see [100] and references therein). These proteins turned out, however, to be related to a family of low molecular weight cytoplasmic proteins (14-16 kD) which include aP2 protein [101] and a fatty acid-binding protein [102] (see also [103] for review) and not to steroid receptors. Both CRBPs (I and II) and CRABPs (I and II) bound with high affinity all-*trans* retinol and all-*trans* RA, respectively. Interestingly, CRABPs do not bind physiologically active 9-*cis* RA [104]. In adult rat tissues CRBP II was primarily expressed in the intestine where it may function in the absorption and/or esterification of retinol [105,106]. CRBP I was found to be more widely expressed and its function may be to store retinol and to facilitate its oxidation [106]. Both in the adult and during development CRABP I and II have been shown to have differential and sometimes non-overlapping patterns of expression, suggesting that they may also have specific functions, perhaps in regulating intracellular concentrations of free all-*trans* RA, its metabolism and/or transport [107-109]. Expression of CRBPs and CRABPs appears to be regulated by retinoids [110-112], possibly providing a regulatory feedback mechanism for a cell to cope with increasing retinoid concentrations. Although it became clear that the above proteins must play important roles in the overall mechanism of vitamin A action, they could not directly affect gene transcription because of their exclusively cytoplasmic localisation (see [103] for review). Furthermore, these proteins appeared to be absent from some cells [103], such as promyelocytic HL-60 cells which were known to undergo granulocytic differentiation when treated with all-*trans* RA [113] and clearly could not be critical for transduction of retinoid signals.

The search for the nuclear mediator of the retinoid action reached its turning point with the discovery of the nuclear receptors for steroid and thyroid hormones, and an understanding that they act as ligand-inducible transcription factors to regulate the transcription of hormone-responsive genes (see [14-16] for reviews). In analogy to other transcription factors, these proteins possessed modular structures which on the basis of amino acid sequence homology could be subdivided into 5 to 6 distinct regions, A-E/F (see [15] and references therein). The most highly conserved (>40% identity across the superfamily) is the C region, which is comprised of 66-68 amino acids and which contains 2 zinc-finger motifs analogous to those found in the DNA-binding-domain (DBD) of the *Xenopus laevis* transcription factor TF-IIIA [114]. Mutagenesis analysis showed that this region of the nuclear receptor indeed constitutes the DBD, which could be further subdivided into the so-called CI and CII functional modules containing the first and second zinc-fingers of the DBD, respectively (see [14,15], next section for further discussion and Fig. 2). In addition to the ligand-binding domain (LBD),

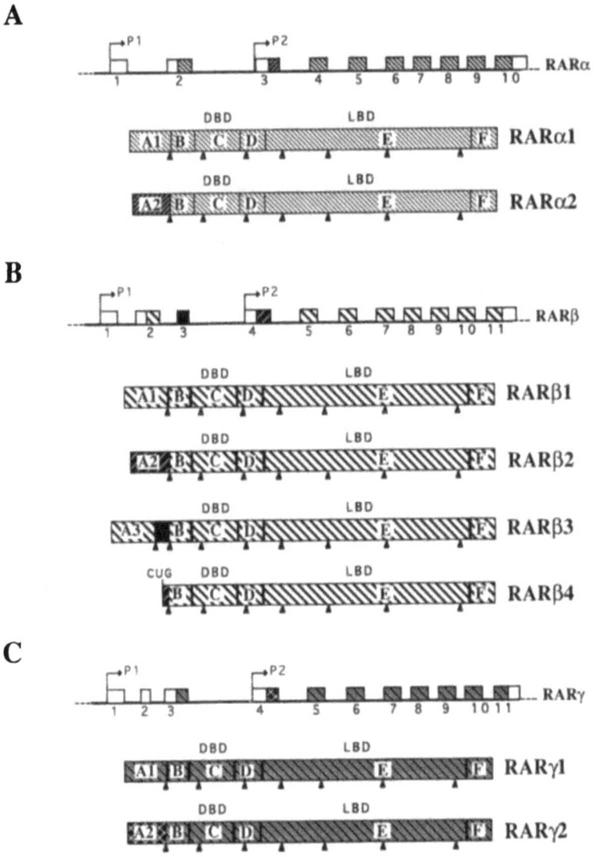

Fig. 1. Schematic representation of the 3 RAR genes and their major isoforms. Exons are represented by shaded boxes and are numbered consecutively. Regions which are not shaded represent 5' and 3' untranslated sequences. Exon/intron structures of RAR-α (A), RAR-ß (B) and RAR-γ (C) genes are as previously described [127,131,213-216]. Note that only exons encoding the major isoforms of the RAR genes are indicated. Two promoters, P1 and P2, in each RAR gene are indicated by broken arrows. Various RAR-α (A), RAR-ß (B) and γ (C) isoforms are indicated by hatched rectangles subdivided into their conserved (B-F) and divergent (A regions) functional domains. Different patterns are used to represent RAR isotype and isoform-specific sequences. Regions encoded by different exons are indicated by arrowheads underneath each diagram. DNA (DBD) and ligand (LBD) binding domains (regions C and E, respectively) are indicated above the scheme for each isoform. Note that this diagram is not essentially drawn to scale.

the E region was found to possess a coiled-coil dimerization interface characterised by multiple heptad repeats of hydrophobic amino acids [115,116] as well as a ligand-dependent transcription activating function (AF-2) [117, 118]. A distinct and ligand-independent transcription activating function (AF-1) was localised to the N-terminal A/B region [119,120]. The activities of both AF-1 and AF-2 were both cell type and promoter specific [117-120]. At the present time the functions of D and F regions are less clear, but they may also possess functions associated with transcriptional regulation [121,122]. Furthermore, the N-terminal amino acids of the D domain are clearly important for specific DNA binding (see Fig. 2 and below).

Exploiting the high degree of sequence conservation between various nuclear receptors, a number of investigators set out to clone new members of this superfamily using degenerate oligonucleotide probes derived from the conserved regions of the DBD sequence. This approach proved very fruitful in the search for the RAR as towards the end of 1987 Giguere et al. [12] and Petkovich et al. [13] reported the cloning of cDNAs encoding the first human RAR, the RAR-α. Shortly afterwards it was recognised that a gene identified from an integration site of the HBV in a single case of hepatocellular carcinoma encodes a second RAR, the RAR-ß [123]. In the process of isolating the mouse homologues of human RARs, another receptor called RAR-γ was identified and its cDNA was cloned [124]. Similar to other members of the nuclear receptor superfamily, the three RARs had structures comprised of 6 regions, A-F (see Fig. 1 for schematic representations). It is worth noting that for each RAR subtype (α, ß, and γ) the sequences of regions A-F are highly conserved between species. In contrast, within a given species only the sequences of regions B, C and E are well conserved and those of regions A, D and F are less so or not at all (see [125] for review). Together with the findings that all 3 RARs have different and tissue-specific patterns of expression [124,126], the above observations suggest that the unique regions of each RAR subtype perform some specific function(s).

To date it has been shown that in the mouse and human, and probably in all vertebrates, three RAR genes exist, each encoding multiple isoforms generated by alternative promoter usage and exon splicing (for review see [125] and references therein). The murine and human RAR genes are very similar in their genomic organisation and structure. Each gene possesses two promoters (P1 and P2) directing expression of at least two major isoforms (α1 and α2, ß1 and ß2, γ1 and γ2) which differ in the sequences encoding their 5'-untranslated regions (5'-utr) and N-terminal A regions, i.e., upstream of the 5' border of the exon encoding the B region (see Fig. 1, A-C). Two additional major RAR-ß isoforms (RAR-ß3 and RAR-ß4) can be generated from the RAR-ß gene by the alternative splicing of transcripts originating from P1 and P2 promoters. The RAR-ß3 differs from RAR-ß1 by an additional 27 amino acids encoded in an exon which is spliced between the exons encoding the A and B regions of RAR-ß1 (see [127] and Fig. 1B). RAR-ß4 on the other hand is generated by alternative splicing of the RAR-ß2 transcript and lacks part of the 5'-utr and nearly the entire A region coding sequence, and its translation starts at a non-AUG codon [128]. Furthermore, the activity of the P2 promoter in each gene is retinoid inducible, and therefore, the RAR-α2, ß2 and ß4, and γ2 expression is regulated by retinoids. The sequences of all the P2 promoters have been cloned and their corresponding retinoic acid response elements (RAREs) characterised (see [129], next section and Fig. 3).

With the exception of the RAR-α1 isoform, whose expression is ubiquitous, all the RARs have been shown to be differentially expressed in the embryo and in adult tissues (for reviews see [109,125,130] and references therein). For example the expression of the mRAR-α2 is low in kidney, muscle heart and skin but high in intestine, liver and lung. RAR-ß1 and ß3 expression is high in the brain whereas the RAR-γ1 isoform is the predominant RAR expressed in skin. The ubiquitous expression of the RAR-α1 isoform is a reflection of the housekeeping nature of the RAR-α P1 promoter which possesses multiple SP1 binding sites, is GC rich and lacks a TATA-box [131]. The fact that every cell in the vertebrate body probably expresses at least the RAR-α1 isoform suggests that functional retinoid-responsive machinery is required in all cells. It is noteworthy from an evolutionary point of view that although all the isoforms have very distinct A region amino acid sequences there is a higher amino acid sequence similarity between the A regions of RAR-α1, ß1 and γ1, (A1 regions) or between those of RAR-α2, ß2 and γ2 (A2 regions) than between the A1 and A2 regions of various RAR isoforms (A1 regions of RAR-α1 and A2 region of RAR-ß2, for example). Furthermore, in all RAR genes the relative order and approximate location of the exons which encode the unique A (A1 and A2) and the common B regions of the two major RAR-α, ß and γ isoforms, are the same (see Fig. 1). Most striking is the sequence identity between the RAR-α2 and ß2 RAREs (see Fig. 3) as well as the adjacent putative regulatory elements which resemble AP-1 binding site and a cAMP response element [127,132]. These structural conservations between various RAR genes indicate that they were all derived by gene and/or chromosome duplication from a single ancestral locus. Nevertheless, due to the variabilities between their A region sequences and their differential patterns of expression, it is reasonable to expect that the above described RAR isoforms will exert some specific functions in the adult organism and/or during development.

In addition to the RARs, another class of nuclear retinoid receptors (retinoid X receptors or RXRs), most closely related to the avian orphan receptor COUP-TF [133] and to the *Drosophila ultraspiracle* gene product [134], was recently discovered [135]. To date 3 different human and mouse RXR genes (α, ß, γ), along with their respective patterns of expression in adult tissues, have been described [136,137]. With the exception of intestine and liver, the RXR-ß was shown to be widely expressed and at higher levels than the other RXR genes. The RXR-α mRNAs were most abundant in the liver and were also detected at lower levels in the kidney, lung, muscle and spleen. The RXR-γ gene on the other hand was found to be expressed at lower levels than the other RXR genes and the highest levels of its expression were detected in the heart and skeletal muscle [137]. In agreement with structures of other nuclear receptors (see above), RXRs were found to possess similar functional domains contained in regions A through E. In contrast to RARs, however, RXRs lacked the F region sequences [129]. Some preliminary results indicate that RXR genes are also expressed as multiple isoforms differing in their N-terminal sequences [129,138,139].

In vitro studies on binding of RARs and TRs to their DNA response elements indicated a requirement of nuclear factors for high affinity binding [140] (see also below and Fig. 4).

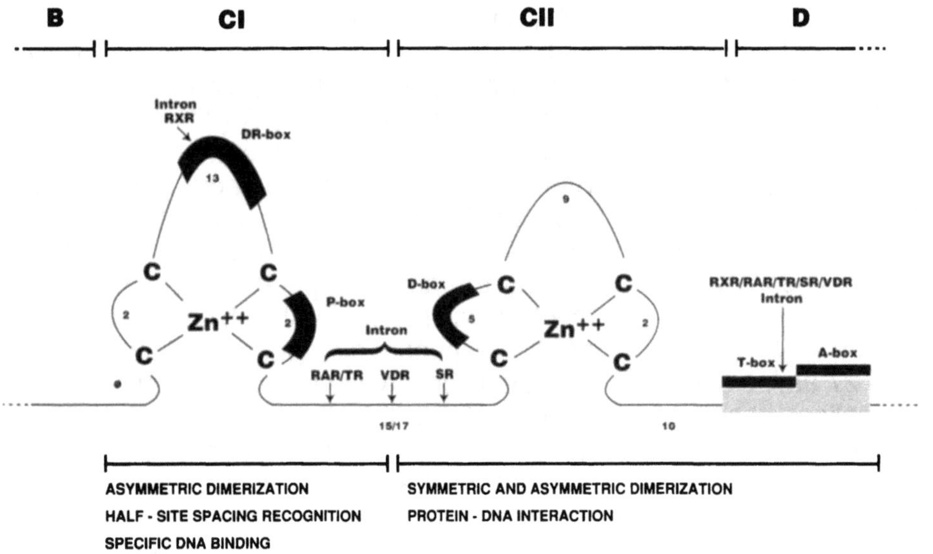

Fig. 2. Schematic representation of a hypothetical structure of the nuclear receptor DBD. Two functional modules CI and CII, as well as their boundaries with B and D regions, are indicated above the diagram. Four conserved cysteines in each module are shown tetrahedrally coordinating the zinc ion (Zn^{++}) to form a "zinc-finger". The numbers denote how many amino acids comprise a given segment between the conserved cysteine residues. Depending on a nuclear receptor, the region between the CI and CII modules can consist of either 15 or 17 amino acids. Positions of introns are indicated with arrows. Note that with the exception of RXR [139], sequences comprising the CI and CII modules in RAR, TR [15], VDR [217] and steroid receptors (SR) [15] are encoded in 2 separate exons. The positions of various functional regions (DR, P, D, T and A boxes) are as indicated. It must be noted that the above functional regions were identified by mutagenesis studies of some but not all of the nuclear receptors. It is likely, however, that these regions are present in the DBDs of all the DR binding (RXR/TR/RAR/VDR subfamily) nuclear receptors.

Subsequently, these factors were identified to be the RXRs (for reviews see [129,141] and references therein). RXRs have also been shown to form functional heterodimers with the vitamin D3 receptor (VDR) [142,143], peroxisome proliferate-activated receptor [144], COUP-FT [145] and *Drosophila ecdysone* receptor [146], indicating the complexity of the nuclear receptor signalling pathways [147]. The natural ligand for the RXRs has been found to be 9-*cis* RA [148,149]. Although the RARs bind both all-*trans* RA and 9-*cis* RA with high affinities, the RXRs have high affinity binding for only the 9-*cis* isomer [104]. In contrast to the RARs, RXRs can homodimerize and bind efficiently to certain RAREs *in vitro* [150], suggesting divergence in the retinoid signalling pathway. Although 9-*cis* RA may enhance the binding of the RXR homodimers to certain response elements (see below), members of the RXR/RAR/TR/VDR subfamily of nuclear receptors do not require a ligand for efficient DNA binding *in vitro* and probably also *in vivo* [151-153].

The ability of RXRs to heterodimerize with a number of different nuclear receptors allows for cross-talk between hormone response pathways. For example, in the presence of 9-*cis* RA and RXR one pathway may be more active than another, therefore, 9-*cis* RA could potentially serve as a physiological switch between different cellular processes (see below). In this respect, it is also worth noting the results of Lehmann et al. [154] who showed that ligand induced formation of RXR homodimers inhibited a thyroid hormone-mediated response. Overexpression of TR, on the other hand, was shown to inhibit RAR-dependent transcriptional activation by titrating out RXR [155]. Likewise, one can expect that the increase in cellular levels of RAR-α2, β2 and γ2 isoforms in response to retinoids may affect the expression of some thyroid hormone and vitamin D3-regulated genes by sequestering the RXR. The extent of such coregulatory interactions will no doubt depend on the relative affinities of various receptors for RXR.

Retinoid Response Elements

In the absence of a natural retinoic acid response element (RARE), all-*trans* RA-dependent transcriptional activation of a reporter gene by the RAR-α was first shown through a so-called 'domain-swap' experiment [156]. Exploiting the modular nature of the nuclear receptors' functional domains Giguere et al. [12] and Petkovich et al. [13] replaced the putative DBD of RAR-α with the DBD from glucocorticoid and oestrogen receptors, respectively, and assayed for the ability of the chimaeric RAR-α proteins to activate transcription in response to all-*trans* RA from either a dexamethasone or oestradiol-responsive promoter. The chimaeric RARs were shown to activate the expression of steroid responsive promoters in an all-*trans* RA-dependent manner, and therefore appeared to function as a nuclear RAR. In the same way the RAR-ß was shown to be responsive to all-*trans* RA, and, interestingly, was found to have apparent ligand binding affinity one order of magnitude higher than RAR-α [123].

Given the high degree of amino acid sequence identity between the DBDs of various members of the nuclear receptor superfamily, it was not surprising to find that the DNA response elements with which they interact were also highly related. Steroid receptors were shown to bind as homodimers to perfect or imperfect palindromic hexanucleotide core-DNA motifs spaced by 3 base pairs. The core recognition sequences for the glucocorticoid and oestrogen receptors were shown to be variants of the AGAACA and AGGTCA motifs, respectively. Initially, the thyroid hormone response elements (TREs) were shown to be similar, or in some cases even identical in sequence to the oestrogen response elements, but would lack spacing between the palindrome half sites. Mutational analyses of glucocorticoid and oestrogen receptors identified amino acids within the first and second zinc fingers of their DBDs which were responsible for recognition of distinct core motifs (P-box) and spacing between the two palindromic half sites (D-box), respectively (see [157, 158] and Fig. 2). Since the P-boxes of TRs and RARs were identical, it was likely that both receptors recognised response elements with very similar core motifs. Working with this hypothesis Umesono et al. [159] have shown that RAR-α could activate transcription from a natural rat growth hormone TRE (imperfect palindrome, TRE_{GH}), or a synthetic palindromic TRE_p, with a core motif AGGTCA and no spacing.

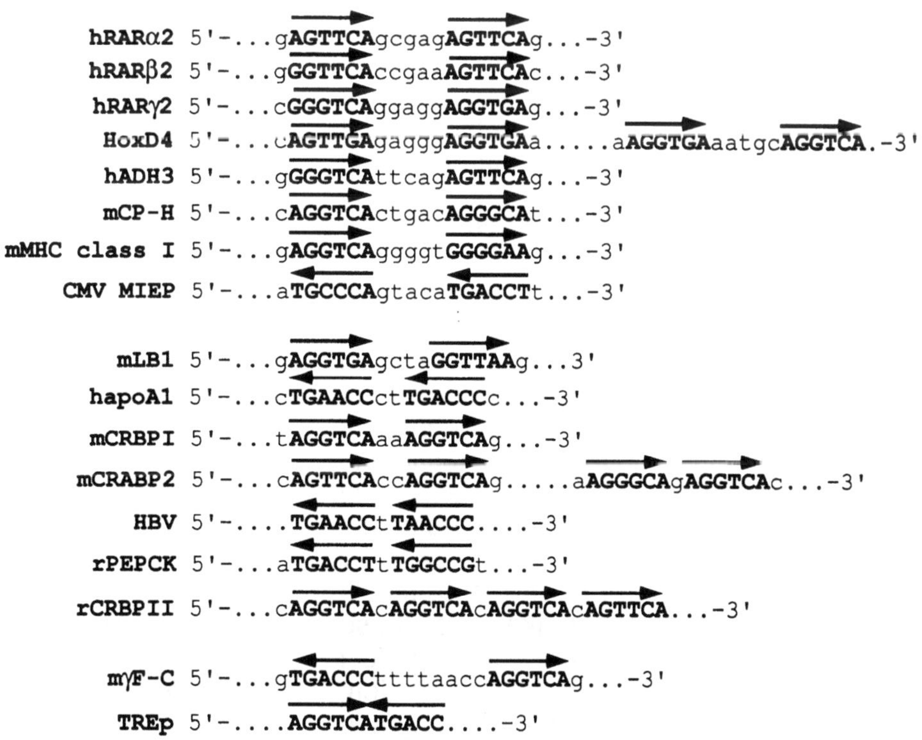

Fig. 3. Various retinoid response elements described to date in a number of human, rodent and viral genes: hRAR-α2, ß2, γ2 - human retinoic acid receptor-α2, ß2, γ2 [132,160,161, 162]; HoxD4 [164]; hADH - human alcohol dehydrogenase [85]; mCP-H - mouse complement factor-H [163]; mMHC class I - mouse major histocompatibility class I [80]; CMV MIEP - cytomegalovirus major immediate-early promoter [94]; mLB1 - mouse laminin B1 [88]; hapoAl - human apolipoprotein AI [165]; mCRBPI - mouse cellular retinol binding protein I [171]; mCRABP II - mouse cellular retinoic acid binding protein II [170]; HBV - hepatitis B virus [97]; rPEPCK - rat phosphoenolpyruvate carboxykinase [86]; rCRBP II- rat cellular retinol binding protein II [112]; mγF-C - mouse γF-crystallin [169]; TREp - synthetic palindromic thyroid hormone response element [159]. Core motifs of each repeat are indicated with capitalised bold letters and their orientation (direct repeat, palindrome or inverted palindrome) is indicated with arrows. The intervening spacer sequences are written with lower case letters.

The first natural RARE was identified in the P2 promoter of the human RAR-ß gene [160,161]. Surprisingly, its sequence lacked dyad symmetry characteristic of palindromic response elements and consisted of an imperfect direct repeat (DR) of a sequence (GGTTCA), which was closely related to the TRE/oestrogen response element core motifs, with an intervening spacing of 5 nucleotides. To date, RAREs consisting of DRs of identical, or closely related, core motifs separated by 5 nucleotides (DR5) have also been identified in the P2 promoters of RAR-α [132] and γ [162] genes, and in the promoters of human alcohol dehydrogenase 3 (hADH3, [85]), mouse complement factor-H (mCP-H, [163]), mouse HoxD4 [164] and mouse major histocompatibility complex class I (mMHC class I [80]) genes as well as in the major immediate-early promoter (MIEP) of human CMV [94] (see Fig. 3). Although heterodimerization with RXRs is required to facilitate efficient binding of RARs to the above RAREs, a RARE preferentially activated by 9-*cis* RA, presumably through ligand-stimulated binding of RXR-α homodimers [150] (see also Fig. 4 for schematic representation), was also identified in the rat CRBP II gene [112] and was shown to consist of 5 direct repeats with a spacing of 1 nucleotide (DR1). Another RXR-specific DR1 RARE (or RXRE) was identified in the HBV enhancer [97]. The so-called site A in the human apolipoprotein AI (hapoAI) gene promoter constitutes a DR2 response element which may selectively bind RXRa/orphan receptor ARP-1 heterodimer [165]. The consensus RARE core motif sequence 5'-(A/G)G(T/G)TCA was derived through comparison of various RAREs and mutagenesis analysis of the RAR-ß2 RARE. It must be noted, however, that not all of the DR motifs conform to this consensus sequence. For example, RAREs from the mCP-H, mMHC class I and human CMV major immediate early promoters display greater degeneracy than allowed by the consensus in one of the two core motifs (see Fig. 3). Although it is likely that these elements indeed function as physiological RAREs, the assays used for their delineation, such as *in vitro* RAR and/or RXR binding and RA-activation of a heterologous promoter in transfected cells, are not physiological. The degree to which these and other RAREs will be bound by RXR/RAR heterodimers or RXR homodimers will no doubt depend on multiple parameters such as the exact sequence of a given RARE (including the spacing sequence), intracellular concentration of the receptors and ligands, and the context of a given promoter (see also below).

Recent studies on differential recognition of a given response element by different nuclear receptors suggested that the spacing between the DRs dictated the extent to which a given element was recognised by the RXR homodimer as well as the RXR/VDR, RXR/TR and RXR/RAR heterodimers [112,166,167]. It was shown that the above combinations of receptor dimers preferentially recognised similar perfect, or degenerate, directly repeated core motifs with spacing of 1, 3 (DR3), 4 (DR4) and 5 nucleotides, respectively (see Fig. 4 for schematic representation); and for example, changing DR3 to DR5 could turn a vitamin D3 response element into a RARE [167]. However, life is not so simple and the 1-3-4-5 rule was found to have many exceptions. For example, RXR/VDR heterodimers were shown to activate the ostiopontin gene expression through a DR3 element, whereas activation of osteocalcin gene expression by vitamin D3 is RXR independent and occurs through a vitamin D3 response element which consists of DR spaced by 6 nucleotides. This activation was suggested to occur through the VDR/VDR homodimer or a heterodimer of the VDR and an unknown nuclear receptor [168]. Furthermore, putative VDR homodimers can also recognise a synthetic palindromic element without spacing and an inverted palindrome with spacing of 12 nucleotides. Recently, Tini et al. [169] also identified a putative RARE in the mouse γF-crystalin (mγF-C) promoter which is an inverted palindrome with 8 nucleotide spacing (see Fig. 3). More importantly to the preceding examples, the RXR/RAR heterodimers have been shown to bind to and activate transcription from natural DR1 and DR2 elements present in the mouse CRABP II promoter [170], and also from DR2 and DR4 elements present in the mouse CRBP I [171] and laminin B1 (mLB1) [88] promoters. A potential DR1 element, which may be recognised by a RXR/RAR heterodimer, appears to mediate all-*trans* RA inducibility of the rat phosphoenolpyruvate carboxykinase (rPEPCK) gene [86]. In fact Mader et al. [172] have shown that RXR/RAR heterodimers bind to DR1 repeats *in vitro* with a higher affinity, albeit with a lesser affinity

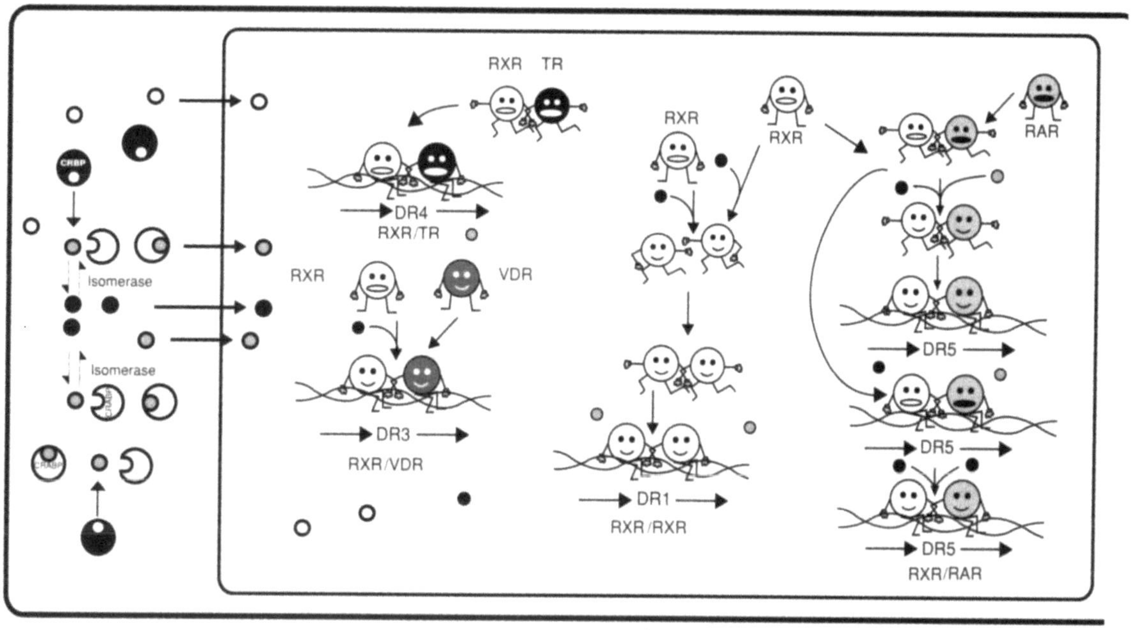

Fig. 4. Cellular components of the retinoid signalling pathway and their interactions. Outer and inner boundaries represent cellular and nuclear membranes, respectively. Retinol, all-*trans* RA and 9-*cis* RA are represented by white, shaded and black circles, respectively. Cytoplasmic retinol and retinoic acid binding proteins are as indicated. CRBP probably functions in oxidation of all-*trans* retinol to all-*trans* RA and CRABP may regulate the cellular levels of free all-*trans* RA. The putative isomerases function in conversion of all-*trans* RA to 9-*cis* RA. Various nuclear receptors are represented by open mouthed (ligand free) and smiling (ligand bound) cartoon characters as indicated. RXR/VDR, RXR/TR and RXR/RAR heterodimers are shown bound to their respective DR3, DR4 and DR5 response elements. RXR homodimers are shown bound to a DR1 repeat. Dimerization between receptors can occur in solution, as indicated for RXR/TR, RXR/RXR and RXR/RAR with subsequent binding of the dimer to a given response element. As shown for RXR/TR and RXR/RAR, ligand-free receptors can probably also bind to their response elements *in vivo*. Homodimerization between RXRs is shown to be stimulated by 9-*cis* RA.

than to other DRs, than did the RXR/RXR homodimers. Nevertheless, preferential binding of the RXR/RXR homodimers to the DR1 RAREs may occur physiologically in cells where RXR and 9-*cis* RA are in excess. Since RXR/RAR heterodimers have much higher affinity for DR5 than for DR1 elements, a much smaller number of these complexes may be sufficient to activate gene expression in the same cell from DR5 elements.

Recent results indicated that, in addition to being dependent on the affinity of the RXR/RAR complex for a given RARE, the magnitude of transcriptional activation by an RXR/RAR heterodimer also depends on the promoter context and the precise nature of the RARE. For example, activation of transcription from the RAR-β2 promoter is highly dependent on RAR AFs; in contrast, AFs of both RXR and RAR contribute equally to activation from the DR1 element in the mCRABP II promoter [170]. Further diversity in the magnitude of retinoid-mediated activation of expression of a specific gene can be generated through the availability of a large number of isoform-specific AF-1s, which can synergise with the ligand-activated AF-2 of the same receptor, or activate transcription on their own independently of AF-2 [173,174]. Promoter and/or cell-type specific combinations of the different parameters described above may physiologically be required to elicit a finely tuned response.

The fact that RAR, RXR, TR and VDR bind as dimers to asymmetrical hormone response elements suggests that their DBDs must possess structural features previously not described for steroid receptors. Indeed a number of recent studies have identified novel functional determinants within the CI module (DR-box) and the very N-terminal sequences of the D region (A and T boxes) (see Fig. 2). The amino acids in the DR-box of the TR, RAR and VDR were shown to constitute an asymmetrical dimerization interface and to be critical for discrimination between different spacing of the DRs [175]. The amino acids in the T and A boxes were shown to mediate additional protein-protein and protein-DNA interactions probably necessary for better recognition of DRs with an appropriate spacing [176,177] and regulation of differential orientations of the DBD [178] on response elements with different symmetries, respectively. Interestingly, in the heterodimeric nuclear receptor complexes which are bound to asymmetrical response elements the RXR always occupies the 5' half of the DR [172,175, 178] (see Fig. 4).

The evolutionary acquisition by nuclear receptors of the ability to heterodimerize clearly increased the diversity of regulatory functions that these factors can mediate. This functional diversification through heterodimerization of transcriptional regulators is not unique to nuclear receptors and can be observed among other families of transcription factors such as members of the Jun-Fos and ATF-CREB families [179,180] as well as myogenic helix-loop-helix proteins [181,182]. It appears that the coevolution of the DBDs of the receptors and the response elements resulted in a very large number of combinatorial possibilities through which a plethora of genes or gene networks could be differentially regulated by a limited number of ligands and nuclear receptors.

Retinoid Receptors and Binding Proteins During Vertebrate Development

The expression of retinoid receptors and cytoplasmic binding proteins has been extensively studied throughout the development of different vertebrates using *in situ* hybridisation. During murine development, the 3 RARs, 2 CRABPs and CRBP I display restricted spatio-temporal patterns of expression [183,184]. In general, the observed spatio-temporal patterns of expression of the above genes correlate well with structures and developmental processes which are affected either by retinoid deficiency or excess. Interestingly, expression of CRBP I and CRABP I correlates with tissues which are most susceptible to the teratogenic effects of retinoid deficiency and excess, respectively (see [109] for review). This association supports the idea that CRBP I may be functioning in the storage of retinol as well as all-*trans* RA biosynthesis and the CRABP I (probably also CRABP II) may regulate the availability of free all-*trans* RA that reaches the nucleus. Since expression of the CRABP II, CRBP I and RAR-ß genes was inducible by all-*trans* RA, the areas of their expression could reflect regions of higher retinoid concentration and/or activity in the embryo. However, the fact that these genes are not expressed in identical patterns indicates a requirement for other cell type and promoter-specific factors for their expression.

During early embryogenesis both the RAR-ß and γ genes are distinctly expressed in the CNS; however, as development progresses the domains of RAR-γ expression became progressively restricted to cartilage and keratinizing squamous epithelia; and therefore, RAR-γ proteins may function in skeletal development and skin morphogenesis. In contrast to RAR-γ, expression of RAR-ß remained in the CNS throughout the later stages of development, and, in addition, became prevalent in mucous secreting epithelia. Expression of the RAR-ß gene could also be observed in the regions of programmed cell death (the interdigital space in the developing limb, for example), suggesting a role for the RAR-ß protein(s) in apoptosis. With the exception of the brain, where the levels of RAR-α transcripts are very low, this gene appears to display an ubiquitous, albeit variable, pattern of expression throughout development (for reviews see [183, 184,109,130]).

Expression of the RXRs during vertebrate development has not been as extensively studied. Nevertheless, limited *in situ* hybridisation data has shown that during avian and mammalian embryogenesis the RXR-γ gene is much more restricted in its pattern of expression than RXR-α and RXR-ß [137,185]. For example, in 16.5 days post-coitum mouse embryos, RXR-γ was primarily expressed in the corpus striatum, pituitary and neck muscle, suggesting that it may have some role in muscle and CNS differentiation. The RXR-α gene was found expressed in various epithelia, but its expression was low in CNS and skeleton. Expression of RXR-α in the intestinal epithelia and other sites of retinoid absorption suggests that this isotype may be active in the regulation of retinoid uptake and storage. The RXR-ß gene, whose expression was ubiquitous, appeared to be the predominant RXR isotype present in the CNS. It is worth noting that the

observation of co-expression of at least one RXR and RAR isotype in every tissue is in agreement with the idea that retinoid signals are transduced by the RXR/RAR heterodimer.
Recent analysis of mice in which either the RAR-α or γ gene was knocked out by homologous recombination in embryonic stem cells, provided direct evidence for a functional role of their products in differentiation of certain tissues as well as in development. However, the generated results are not without some surprises, since the loss of both alleles of a given receptor was less detrimental than that which might have been expected from the pattern of its expression. For example, RAR-α gene knockout [186] resulted in homozygotes which at birth showed no obvious malformation but displayed significantly lower survival rates compared with heterozygous or wild type animals. Mutant animals which survived for longer time periods appeared normal except that the males were sterile due to testes degeneration. Furthermore, knockout of the RAR-α1 isoform produced no phenotype [186,187]. Given the ubiquitous nature of RAR-α1 expression, this result was rather surprising and suggested that the processes disrupted in the RAR-α mutant animals are largely mediated by the RAR-α2 isoform. Mice homozygous for RAR-γ gene knockout [188] displayed a more severe phenotype than the RAR-α null homozygotes. These animals exhibited growth deficiency, early lethality and male sterility. Importantly, some of the abnormalities seen in the RAR-γ mutant mice, such as squamous metaplasia of seminal vesicles and prostate, were identical to defects observed in offspring of animals fed on a vitamin A-deficient diet. Lack of expression of the RAR-γ gene also led to an antero-posterior homeotic transformation of the vertebrae. Together with observations that some skeletal malformations induced by excess all-*trans* RA did not occur in the RAR-γ null foetuses, the results reported by Lohnes et al. [188] prove that RAR-γ proteins are directly involved in transduction of at least some of the retinoid signals. Analogously to the observation with RAR-α1, however, lack of expression of RAR-γ2 isoform did not produce any phenotype which could be observed in laboratory animals without examination of a very large number of mice [188]. The apparent functional redundancy between the RAR isoforms is not unique to the RARs but is often observed within other families of developmentally important transcription factors [189,190]. The presence of a number of redundant RAR isoforms may be of functional importance during evolution. For example, with time these redundant molecules may acquire specific functions required to meet novel selective pressures. Generation of mice which lack expression of additional RARs, RXRs, and cellular retinoid binding proteins, as well as mice in which multiple genes have been disrupted, will be most useful in elucidating specific roles for these molecules during development and/or in the adult organism.

Cross-Talk Between Retinoid and Cell Membrane Receptor Signalling Pathways

As mentioned above, retinoids regulate the expression of a number of genes which are key components of cell membrane signalling pathways. An important example which demonstrates a different level of cross-talk between these signalling pathways is the ability of all-*trans* RA to inhibit AP-1 activity and hence negatively regulate the expression of AP-1 responsive genes such as collagenase and stromelysin [82,191-193]. AP-1 activity, which consists of dimeric protein complexes between members of the Fos and Jun families of transcription factors, has been implicated in transduction of cell membrane generated signals at the level of the transcriptional regulation of gene expression. The effect of all-*trans* RA on AP-1 activity was shown to be independent of the DNA binding by the RARs and to depend solely on protein-protein interactions between the RARs and the c-Jun component of AP-1 [192,193]. Conversely, an interaction between AP-1 and RAR proteins could also inhibit RAR activity. Since retinoid and AP-1 activities have been associated with opposing effects on cellular proliferation, proper interaction and balance between these distinct signalling pathways are probably necessary for normal cellular growth; their loss or deregulation may be implicated in tumorigenesis (see below).
Another potential way in which cell membrane-mediated signalling could interact with retinoid signal transduction is through receptor phosphorylation. RARs have been demonstrated to undergo phosphorylation *in vivo* [194-196],

and recently Huggenvik et al. [197] demonstrated ligand-independent transcriptional activation by RAR which may be dependent on its phosphorylation by protein kinase A. This potential relationship between phosphorylation by a protein kinase and activation of a nuclear receptor is reflected also in recent studies showing that dopamine can activate steroid receptors, presumably through cell membrane mediating signalling [198].

Role of Retinoid Receptors in Tumorigenesis

Given their role in the control of the cellular growth and proliferation, it is not surprising that some nuclear receptors have turned out to be protooncogenes [199,200]. For example, the oncogenic form of the TR, v-erbA oncogene present in the avian erythroblastosis virus, acts in a dominant negative fashion to inhibit expression of genes associated with erythroid differentiation and hence blocks thyroid hormone-dependent erythropoiesis [151,201]. Interestingly, the ability of the v-erbA oncoprotein to transform haemopoietic cells has been correlated with its ability to suppress the retinoid response [202]. It has been suggested that one of the possible mechanisms by which v-erbA can participate in leukaemogenesis is the abrogation of the inactivation of AP-1 activity by RARs and TRs [203]. Furthermore, in acute promyelocytic leukaemia the RAR-α gene was found to be translocated to either of two distinct chromosomal loci, PML or PLZF, and the resulting chimaeric PML- and PLZF-RAR-α proteins are thought to function in leukaemogenesis, perhaps in a dominant negative manner analogous to the v-erbA oncogene (for reviews see [204-206] and references therein). RAR-β gene disruption may also prove to be an important factor in tumorigenesis as this gene is abnormally expressed in a number of lung cancer cell lines and tissues [207,208]. Additionally, in a single case of hepatocellular carcinoma, the RAR-β gene was found to be the site of HBV integration [209]. Although the presence of chimaeric HBV-RAR-β fusion proteins was not determined due to unavailability of patient material, genetically engineered HBV pre-S antigen-RAR-β chimaeric protein was shown to transform avian erythroid progenitors [210].

Concluding Remarks

It is clear that in the past 7 years remarkable progress has been made in identifying the molecular components of the retinoid signalling pathways and understanding the mechanisms through which retinoids exert their highly pleiotropic effects. As perhaps anticipated, these mechanisms are very complex and involve a large number of interacting molecules whose combinatorial and concerted actions at the level of regulation of gene expression elicit specific physiological responses. The precise nature of retinoid signals and responses in a given cell most likely depends on multiple cell type-specific parameters such as intracellular levels of free retinoids (probably dependent on the relative levels of biosynthetic and catabolic enzymes as well as CRBPs and CRABPs); concentrations of various retinoid receptors and their isoforms as well as nuclear receptors which can compete for the common heterodimerization partner - RXR; and lastly the exact nature of cell type-specific transcription factors bound to given promoter and/or enhancer elements containing relevant RAREs. One unresolved question in this field is whether retinoids can exert any effects independently of the nuclear retinoid receptors. Retinoylation of intracellular proteins has been proposed to be one such a mechanism [211], however, there is a lack of any functional significance to this phenomenon. Recently, 14-hydroxy-4,14-*retro*-retinol has been shown to be required for B-lymphocyte proliferation and survival [212]. The authors claimed that this retinoid did not bind to retinoid receptors and suggested that it may mediate its effects through a different mechanism. Nevertheless, it is not entirely clear whether this retinoid is not metabolised to an active derivative which could mediate effects through binding to RARs and/or RXRs. Additionally, at the present time the possible existence of as yet unknown nuclear retinoid receptors, which may bind 14-hydroxy-4,14-*retro*-retinol, cannot be excluded. It therefore appears that most of the retinoid effects on cellular growth and differentiation as well as during development can be accounted for by the mechanisms involving the action of retinoid receptors. The final resolution of the above and many other questions still lies in the future. The high degree of complexity and diversity of interactions within the retinoid family of nuclear receptors as well as between the retinoid and other signalling pathways will no doubt keep many scientists in the retinoid field busy for many years to come.

Acknowledgements

I am grateful to Drs N. Brand, L. Wiedemann and A. Lloyd as well as J. Davies and P. Strutt for critical reading of the manuscript. I am also grateful to the Leukaemia Research Fund of Great Britain and the National Institutes of Health for support.

List of Abbreviations

AF	activating function
CMV	cytomegalovirus
CNS	central nervous system
CRABP	cellular retinoic acid binding protein
CRBP	cellular retinol binding protein
DBD	DNA binding domain
DR	direct repeat
hADH3	human alcohol dehydrogenase 3
hapoA1	human apolipoprotein A1
HBV	hepatitis B virus
LBD	ligand binding domain
mCP-H	mouse complement factor-H
mγFC	mouse γF-crystallin
MIEP	major immediate early promoter
mLB1	mouse laminin B1
mMHC	mouse major histocompatibility complex
PGF	peptide growth factor
PML	promyelocytic leukaemia gene
PLZF	promyelocytic leukaemia zinc finger gene
RA	retinoic acid
RAR	retinoic acid receptor
RARE	retinoic acid response element
rPEPCK	rat phosphoenolpyruvate carboxykinase
RXR	retinoid X receptor
TGF-ß	transforming growth factor-ß
TR	thyroid hormone receptor
TRE	thyroid hormone response element
VDR	vitamin D3 receptor
ZPA	zone of polarising activity

REFERENCES

1 McCollum EV and Davis M: The necessity of certain lipins in the diet during growth. J Biol Chem 1913 (15):167-175

2 Bloch CE: Blindness and other diseases in children arising from deficient nutrition (lack of soluble A factor). Am J Dis Child 1924 (27):139-148

3 Wolbach SB and Howe PR: Tissue changes following deprivation of fat-soluble A vitamin. J Exp Med 1925 (42):753-777

4 Wilson JG, Roth CB and Warkany J: An analysis of the syndrome of malformations induced by maternal vitamin A deficiency. Effects of restoration of vitamin A at various times during gestation. Am J Anat 1953 (92):189-217

5 Kalter H and Warkany J: Experimental production of congenital malformations in mammals by metabolic procedure. Physiol Rev 1959 (39):69-115

6 Thompson JN, Howell JM and Pitt GAJ: Vitamin A and reproduction in rats. Proc R Soc Lond (B) 1964 (159):510-535

7 Moore T: Effects of vitamin A deficiency in animals: pharmacology and toxicology of vitamin A. In: Sebrell WH and Harris RS (eds) The Vitamins. Academic Press, New York 1967 pp 245-266

8 Sporn MB, Roberts AB and Goodman DS: Retinoids. Vol 1 and 2. Academic Press, Orlando, Florida 1984

9 Livrea MA and Packer L: Retinoids. Marcel Dekker, New York 1993

10 Ross AC: Cellular metabolism and activation of retinoids: roles of cellular retinoid-binding proteins. FASEB J 1993 (7):317-327

11 Wald G: Molecular basis of visual excitations. Science 1968 (162):230-239

12 Giguere V, Ong ES, Segui P and Evans RM: Identification of a receptor for the morphogen retinoic acid. Nature 1987 (330):624-629

13 Petkovich M, Brand NJ, Krust A and Chambon P: A human retinoic acid receptor which belongs to the family of nuclear receptors. Nature 1987 (330):444-450

14 Evans RM: The steroid and thyroid hormone receptor super-family. Science 1988 (240):889-895

15 Green S and Chambon P: Nuclear receptors enhance our understanding of transcription regulation. Trends Genet 1988 (4):309-314

16 Beato M: Gene regulation by steroid hormones. Cell 1989 (56):335-344

17 Mori S: The changes in the para-ocular glands which follow the administration of diets low in fat-soluble A, with notes of the effect of the same diets on the salivary glands and the mucosa of the larynx and trachea. Johns Hopkins Hosp Bull 1922 (33):357-359

18 Asselineau D, Bernard BA, Bailly C and Darmon M: Retinoic acid improves epidermal morphogenesis. Dev Biol 1989 (133):322-335

19 Smith MA, Parkinson DR, Cheson BD and Friedman MA: Retinoids in cancer therapy. J Clin Onc 1992 (10):839-864

20 Peck GL: Synthetic retinoids in dermatology. In: Sporn MB, Roberts AB and Goodman DS (eds) The Retinoids. Academic Press, Orlando 1984 pp 391-411

21 Lotan R: Effects of vitamin A and its analogs (retinoids) on normal and neoplastic cells. Biochim Biophys Acta 1980 (605):33-91

22 Roberts AB and Sporn MB: Cellular biology and biochemistry of the retinoids. In: Sporn MB, Roberts AB and Goodman DS (ed) The Retinoids. Academic Press, Orlando, Florida 1984 pp 209-284

23 Hodges RE, Sauberlich HE, Canham JE, Wallace DL, Rucker RB, Mejia LA and Mohanram M: Hematopoietic studies in vitamin A deficiency. Am J Clin Nutr 1978 (31):876-885

24 Amatruda T and Koeffler H: Retinoids and cells of the hematopoietic system. In: Sherman M (ed) Retinoids and Cell Differentiation. CRC Press, Boca Raton, Florida 1986 pp 79-103

25 Ross AC: Vitamin A status: relationship to immunity and the antibody response. Proc Soc Exp Biol Med 1992 (200):303-320

26 Yang Y, Vacchio MS and Ashwell JD: 9-*cis*-retinoic acid inhibits activation-driven T-cell apoptosis: Implications for retinoid X receptor involvement in thymocyte development. Proc Natl Acad Sci USA 1993 (90):6170-6174

27 Kochhar DM: Teratogenic activity of retinoic acid. Acta Pathol Microbiol Scand 1961 (70):398-404

28 Morriss GM and Thorogood PV: An approach to cranial neural crest cell migration and differentiation in mammalian embryos. In: Johnson MH (ed) Development in Mammals. Elsevier North-Holland, Amsterdam 1978 pp 363-411

29 Kochhar DM: Limb development in mouse embryos 1. Analysis of teratogenic effects of retinoic acid. Teratology 1973 (7):289-298

30 Webster WS, Johnston MC, Lammer EJ and Sulik KK: Isotretinoin embryopathy and the cranial neural crest; an in vivo and in vitro study. J Craniofac Genet Dev Biol 1986 (6):211-222

31 Sulik KK, Cook CS and Webster WS: Teratogens and craniofacial malformations; relationships to cell death. Development 1988 (103 suppl):213-232

32 Alles AJ and Sulik KK: Retinoic acid induced limb-reduction defects: perturbation of zones of programmed cell death as a pathogenetic mechanism. Teratology 1989 (40):163-171

33 Eichele G: Retinoids and vertebrate limb pattern formation. Trends Genet 1989 (5):246-251

34 Tabin CJ: Retinoids, homeoboxes, and growth factors: toward molecular models for limb development. Cell 1991 (66):199-217

35 Saunders JW and Gasseling MT: Ectoderm-mesenchymal interactions in the origin of wing symmetry. In: Fleischmajer R and Billingham RE (eds) Epithelial-Mesenchymal Interactions. Williams and Wilkins, Baltimore 1968 pp 78-97

36 Tickle C, Summerbell D and Wolpert L: Positional signalling and specification of digits in chick limb morphogenesis. Nature 1975 (254):199-202

37 Niazi IA and Saxena S: Inhibitory and modifying influence of excess of vitamin A on tail regeneration in Bufo tadpoles. Experientia 1968 (24):852-853
38 Niazi IA and Saxena S: Abnormal hind limb regeneration in tadpoles of the toad, *Bufo andersoni*, exposed to excess vitamin A. Folia Biol (Krakow) 1978 (26):3-11
39 Tickle C, Alberts BM, Wolpert L and Lee J: Local application of retinoic acid to the limb bud mimics the action of the polarizing region. Nature 1982 (296):564-565
40 Thaller C and Eichele G: Identification and spatial distribution of retinoids in the developing chick limb bud. Nature 1987 (327):625-628
41 Thaller C and Eichele G: Isolation of 3,4-didehydroretinoic acid, a novel morphogenetic signal in the chick wing bud. Nature 1990 (345): 815-819
42 Thaller C, Hoffmann C and Eichele G: 9-*cis*-retinoic acid, a potent inducer of digit pattern duplications in the chick wing bud. Development 1993 (118):957-965
43 Slack JMW: We have a morphogen! Nature 1987 (327):553-554
44 Brockes J: We may not have a morphogen. Nature 1991 (350):15
45 Wanek N, Gardiner DM, Muneoka K and Bryant SV: Conversion by retinoic acid of anterior cells into ZPA cells in the chick wing bud. Nature 1991 (350):81-83
46 Noji S, Nohno T, Koyama E, Muto K, Ohyama K, Aoki Y, Tamura K, Ohsugl K, Ide H, Taniguchi S and Saito T: Retinoic acid induces polarizing activity but is unlikely to be a morphogen in the chick limb bud. Nature 1991 (350):83-86
47 Riddle RD, Johnson RL, Laufer E and Tabin C: *Sonic hedgehog* mediates the polarizing activity of the ZPA. Cell 1993 (75):1401-1416
48 Maden M: Vitamin A and pattern formation in the regenerating limb. Nature 1982 (295):672-675
49 Summerbell D and Maden M: Retinoic acid, a developmental signalling molecule. Trends Neurosci 1990 (13):142-147
50 Durston AJ, Timmermans JPM, Hage WJ, Hendriks HFJ, de Vries NJ, Heideveld M and Nieuwkoop PD: Retinoic acid causes an anteroposterior transformation in the developing central nervous system. Nature 1989 (340):140-144
51 Sive HL, Draper BW, Harland RM and Weintraub H: Identification of a retinoic acid-sensitive period during primary axis formation in *Xenopus laevis*. Genes Dev 1990 (4):932-942
52 Pijnappel WWM, Hendriks HFJ, Folkers GE, van den Brink CE, Dekker EJ, Edelenbosch C, van der Saag PT and Durston AJ: The retinoid ligand 4-oxo-retinoic acid is a highly active modulator of positional specification. Nature 1993 (366):340-344
53 Wagner M, Thaller C, Jessell T and Eichele G: Polarizing activity and retinoid synthesis in the floor plate of the neural tube. Nature 1990 (345): 819-822
54 Hogan BLM, Thaller C and Eichele G: Evidence that Hensen's node is a site of retinoic acid synthesis. Nature 1992 (359):237-241
55 Chen YP and Solursh M: Retinoic acid can induce secondary axis formation in the chick embryo. J Cell Biol 1990 (111):236A
56 Kessel M and Gruss P: Homeotic transformations of murine vertebrae and concomitant alteration of *hox* codes induced by retinoic acid. Cell 1991 (67):89-104
57 Boncinelli E, Simeone A, Acampora D and Mavilio F: HOX gene activation by retinoic acid. Trends Genet 1991 (7):329-334
58 Duboule D: Patterning in the vertebrate limb. Current Opinion in Genetics and Development 1991 (1):211-216
59 Kessel M, Bailing R and Gruss P: Variations of cervical vertebrae after expression of a *Hox 1.1* transgene in mice. Cell 1990 (61):301-308
60 Lufkin T, Dierich A, LeMeur M, Mark M and Chambon P: Disruption of the *Hox-1.6* homeobox gene results in defects in a region corresponding to its rostral domain of expression. Cell 1991 (66):1105-1119
61 Rijli F, Mark M, Lakkaraju S, Dierich A, Dolle P and Chambon P: A homeotic transformation is generated in the rostral branchial region of the head by disruption of *Hoxa-2*, which acts as a selector gene. Cell 1993 (75):1333-1349
62 Morgan BA, Ipisua-Belmonte J-C, Duboule D and Tabin CJ: Targeted misexpression of *Hox-4.6* in the avian limb bud causes apparent homeotic transformations. Nature 1992 (358):236-239
63 Scott MP: Vertebrate homeobox gene nomenclature. Cell 1992 (71):551-553
64 McGinnis W and Krumlauf R: Homeobox genes and axial patterning. Cell 1992 (68):283-382
65 Mavilio F: Regulation of vertebrate homeobox-containing genes by morphogens. Eur J Biochem 1993 (212):273-288
66 Kessel M: Respecification of vertebral identities by retinoic acid. Development 1992 (115):487-501
67 Izpisua-Belmonte J-C, Tickle C, Dolle P, Wolpert L and Duboule D: Expression of the homeobox *Hox-4* genes and the specification of position in chick wing development. Nature 1991 (350):585-589
68 Ruiz i Altaba A and Melton DA: Interaction between peptide growth factors and homeobox genes in the establishment of antero-posterior polarity in frog embryos. Nature 1989 (341):33-38
69 Green JB and Smith JC: Growth factors as morphogens: do gradients and thresholds establish body plan? Trends Genet 1991 (7):245-250
70 Cho KWY and De Robertis EM: Differential activation of *Xenopus* homeo box genes by mesoderm-inducing growth factors and retinoic acid. Genes Dev 1990 (4):1910-1916
71 Roberts AB and Sporn MB: Mechanistic interrelationships between two superfamilies: The steroid/retinoid receptors and transforming growth factor-ß. In: Parker MG (ed) Cancer Surveys Vol 14: Growth Regulation by Nuclear Hormone Receptors. Cold Spring Harbor Laboratory Press, 1992 pp 205-220

72 Schöler HR: Octamania: The POU factors in murine development. Trends Genet 1991 (7):323-328
73 Gruss P and Walther C: Pax in development. Cell 1992 (69):719-722
74 El-Baradi T and Pieler T: Zinc finger proteins: what we know and what we would like to know. Mech Dev 1991 (35):155-169
75 Darland T, Samuels M, Edwards SA, Sukhatme VP and Adamson ED: Regulation of Egr-1 (Zfp-6) and c-*fos* expression in differentiating embryonal carcinoma cells. Oncogene 1991 (6):1367-1376
76 Rosner MH, Vigano MA, Ozato K, Timmons PM, Poirier F, Rigby PWJ and Staudt LM: A POU-domain transcription factor in early stem cells and germ cells of the mammalian embryo. Nature 1990 (345):686-692
77 Sham MH, Vesque C, Nonchev S, Marshall H, Frain M, Das Gupta R, Whiting J, Wilkinson D, Charnay P and Krumlauf R: The zinc finger gene *Krox20* regulates *HoxB2 (Hox2.8)* during hindbrain segmentation. Cell 1993 (72):183-196
78 Chytil F and Riaz-ul-Haq: Vitamin A mediated gene expression. Critical Reviews in Eukaryotic Gene Expression 1990 (1):61-73
79 Lüscher B, Mitchell PJ, Williams T and Tijan R: Regulation of transcription factor AP-2 by the morphogen retinoic acid and by second messengers. Genes Dev 1989 (3):1507-1517
80 Segars JH, Nagata T, Bours V, Medin JA, Franzoso G, Blanco JCG, Drew PD, Becker KG, An J, Tang T, Stephany DA, Neel B, Siebenlist U and Ozato K: Retinoic acid induction of major histocompatibility complex class I genes in NT-era-2 embryonal carcinoma cells involves induction of NF-κB (p50-p65) and retinoic acid receptor ß-retinoid X receptor ß heterodimers. Mol Cell Biol 1993 (13):6157-6169
81 Wang C, Kelly J, Bowen-Pope DF and Stiles CD: Retinoic acid promotes transcription of the platelet-derived growth factor α-receptor gene. Mol Cell Biol 1990 (10):6781-6784
82 Nicholson RC, Mader S, Nagpal S, Leid M, Rochette-Egly C and Chambon P: Negative regulation of the rat stromelysin gene promoter by retinoic acid is mediated by an AP1 binding site. EMBO J 1990 (9):4443-4454
83 Husmann M, Gorgen I, Weisgerber C and Bitter-Suermann D: Up-regulation of embryonic NCAM in an EC cell line by retinoic acid. Dev Biol 1989 (136):194-200
84 Bentley D and Groudine M: A block to elongation is largely responsible for decreased transcription of c-*myc* in differentiated HL60 cells. Nature 1986 (321):702-706
85 Duester G, Shean ML, McBride MS and Stewart MJ: Retinoic acid response element in the human alcohol dehydrogenase gene *ADH3* implications for regulation of retinoic acid synthesis. Mol Cell Biol 1991 (11):1638-1646
86 Hall RK, Scott DK, Noisin EL, Lucas PC and Granner DK: Activation of the phosphoenolpyruvate carboxykinase gene retinoic acid response element is dependent on a retinoic acid receptor/coregulator complex. Mol Cell Biol 1992 (12):5527-5535
87 Stellmach V, Leask A and Fuchs E: Retinoid-mediated transcriptional regulation of keratin genes in human epidermal and squamous cell carcinoma cells. Proc Natl Acad Sci USA 1991 (88):4582-4586
88 Vasios G, Mader S, Gold JD, Leid M, Lutz Y, Gaub MP, Chambon P and Gudas L: The late retinoic acid induction of laminin B1 gene transcription involves RAR binding to the responsive element. EMBO J 1991 (10):1149-1158
89 Hirsch MR, Gaugler L, Deagostini-Bazin H, Bally-Cuif L and Goridis C: Identification of positive and negative regulatory elements governing cell-type-specific expression of the neural cell adhesion molecule gene. Mol Cell Biol 1990 (10):1959-1968
90 Kopan R and Fuchs E: A new look into an old problem: keratins as tools to investigate determination, morphogenesis, and differentiation in skin. Genes Dev 1989 (3):1-15
91 Choi Y and Fuchs E: TGF-ß and retinoic acid: regulators of growth and modifiers of differentiation in human epidermal cells. Cell Regulation 1990 (1):791-809
92 Bartsch D, Boye B, Baust C, zur Hausen H and Schwarz E: Retinoic acid-mediated repression of human papillomavirus 18 transcription and different ligand regulation of the retinoic acid receptor ß gene in non-tumorigenic and tumorigenic HeLa hybrid cells. EMBO J 1992 (11):2283-2291
93 Poli G, Kinter AL, Justement JS, Bressler P, Kehrl JH and Fauci AS: Retinoic acid mimics transforming growth factor ß in the regulation of human immunodeficiency virus expression in monocytic cells. Proc Natl Acad Sci USA 1992 (89):2689-2693
94 Ghazal P, DeMattei C, Giulietti E, Kliewer SA, Umesono K and Evans RM: Retinoic acid receptors initiate induction of the cytomegalovirus enhancer in embryonal cells. Proc Natl Acad Sci USA 1992 (89):7630-7634
95 Sista ND, Pagano JS, Liao W and Kenney S: Retinoic acid is a negative regulator of the Epstein-Barr virus protein (BZLF1) that mediates disruption of latent infection. Proc Natl Acad Sci USA 1993 (90):3894-3898
96 Bolander FF Jr and Blackstone ME: Thyroid hormone requirement for retinoic acid induction of mouse mammary tumor virus expression. J Virol 1990 (64):5192-5193
97 Huan B and Siddiqui A: Retinoid X receptor RXRα binds to and trans-activates the hepatitis B virus enhancer. Proc Natl Acad Sci USA 1992 (89):9059-9063
98 Jensen EV and DeSombre ER: Mechanism of action of the female sex hormones. Annu Rev Biochem 1972 (41):203-230
99 Bashor MM, Toft DO and Chytil F: In vitro binding of retinol to rat-tissue components. Proc Natl Acad Sci USA 1973 (70):3483-3487
100 Chytil F and Stump DG: Cellular retinoic acid- and retinol-binding proteins. In: Saurat JH (ed) Retinoids: 10 Years On. Karger, Basel 1991 pp 38-45

101 Hunt CR, Ro JH-S, Dobson DE, Min HY and Spiegelman BM: Adipocyte P2 gene: Developmental expression and homology of 5'-flanking sequences among fat cell-specific genes. Proc Natl Acad Sci USA 1986 (83):3786-3790

102 Sweetser DA, Lowe JB and Gorden JI: The nucleotide sequence of the rat liver fatty acid-binding protein gene. J Biol Chem 1986 (261): 5553-5561

103 Chytil F and Ong D: Cellular retinoid-binding proteins. In: Sporn MB, Roberts AB and Goodman DS (eds) The Retinoids. Vol 2. Academic Press, Orlando 1984 pp 90-123

104 Allenby G, Bocquel M-T, Saunders M, Kazmer S, Speck J, Rosenberger M, Lovey A, Kastner P, Grippo JF, Chambon P and Levin AA: Retinoic acid receptors and retinoid X receptors: Interactions with endogenous retinoic acids. Proc Natl Acad Sci USA 1993 (90):30-34

105 Li E, Demmer LA, Sweetser DA, Ong DE and Gordon JI: Rat cellular retinol-binding protein II: use of a cloned cDNA to define its primary structure, tissue-specific expression, and developmental regulation. Proc Natl Acad Sci USA 1986 (83):5779-5783

106 Levin MS, Li E, Ong DE and Gordon JI: Comparison of the tissue-specific expression and developmental regulation of two closely linked rodent genes encoding cytosolic retinol-binding proteins. J Biol Chem 1987 (262):7118-7124

107 Blomhoff R, Green MH, Berg T and Norum KR: Transport and storage of vitamin A. Science 1990 (250):399-404

108 Lohnes D, Dierich A, Ghyselinck N, Kastner P, Lampron C, LeMeur M, Lufkin T, Mendelsohn C, Nakshatri H and Chambon P: Retinoid receptors and binding proteins. J Cell Sci 1992 (16):69-76

109 Morriss-Kay G: Retinoic acid and craniofacial development: molecules and morphogenesis. BioEssays 1993 (15):9-15

110 Wei L-N, Blaner WS, Goodman DS and Nguyen-Huu MC: Regulation of the cellular retinoid-binding proteins and their messenger ribonucleic acids during P19 embryonal carcinoma cell differentiation induced by retinoic acid. Mol Endocrinol 1989 (3):454-463

111 Giguere V, Lyn S, Yip P, Siu C-H and Amin S: Molecular cloning of cDNA encoding a second cellular retinoic acid-binding protein. Proc Natl Acad Sci USA 1990 (87):6233-6237

112 Mangelsdorf DJ, Umesono K, Kliewer SA, Borgmeyer U, Ong ES and Evans RM: A direct repeat in the cellular retinol-binding protein type II gene confers differential regulation by RXR and RAR. Cell 1991 (66):555-561

113 Breitman TR, Selonick SE and Collins SJ: Induction of differentiation of the human promyelocytic leukemia cell line (HL-60) by retinoic acid. Proc Natl Acad Sci USA 1980 (77):2936-2940

114 Miller J, McLachlan AD and Klug A: Repetitive zinc-binding domains in the protein transcription factor IIIA from *Xenopus* oocytes. EMBO J 1985 (4):1609-1614

115 Fawell SE, Lees JA, White R and Parker MG: Characterization and colocalization of steroid binding and dimerization activities in the mouse estrogen receptor. Cell 1990 (60):953-962

116 Forman BM, Yang C-r, Au M, Casanova J, Ghysdael J and Samuels HH: A domain containing leucine-zipper-like motifs mediate novel in vivo interactions between the thyroid hormone and retinoic acid receptors. Mol Endocrinol 1989 1610-1676

117 Tora L, White J, Brou C, Tasset D, Webster N, Scheer E and Chambon P: The human estrogen receptor has two independent non-acidic transcriptional activation functions. Cell 1989 (59):477-487

118 Tasset D, Tora L, Fromental C, Scheer E and Chambon P: Distinct classes of transcriptional activating domains function by different mechanisms. Cell 1990 (62):1177-1187

119 Tora L, Gronemeyer H, Turcotte B, Gaub MP and Chambon P: The N-terminal region of the chicken progesterone receptor specifies target gene activation. Nature 1988 (333):185-188

120 Tora L, Gaub M-P, Mader S, Dierich A, Bellard M and Chambon P: Cell-specific activity of a GGTCA half-palindromic oestrogen-responsive element in the chicken ovalbumin gene promoter. EMBO J 1988 (7):3771-3778

121 Baniahmad A, Kohne AC and Renkawitz R: A transferable silencing domain is present in the thyroid hormone receptor, in the v-erbA oncogene product and in the retinoic acid receptor. EMBO J 1992 (11):1015-1023

122 Lee Y and Mahdavi V: The D domain of the thyroid hormone receptor $\alpha 1$ specifies positive and negative transcriptional regulation functions. J Biol Chem 1993 (268):2021-2028

123 Brand N, Petkovich M, Krust A, Chambon P, de Thé H, Marchio A, Tiollais P and Dejean A: Identification of a second human retinoic acid receptor. Nature 1988 (332):850-853

124 Zelent A, Krust A, Petkovich M, Kastner P and Chambon P: Cloning of murine α and ß retinoic acid receptors and a novel receptor γ predominantly expressed in skin. Nature 1989 (339):714-717

125 Chambon P, Zelent A, Petkovich M, Mendelsohn C, Leroy P, Krust A, Kastner P and Brand N: The family of retinoic acid nuclear receptors. In: Saurat J-H (ed) Retinoids: 10 Years On. S Karger, Basel 1991 pp 10-27

126 de Thé H, Marchio A, Tiollais P and Dejean A: Differential expression and ligand regulation of the retinoic acid receptor α and ß genes. EMBO J 1989 (8):429-433

127 Zelent A, Mendelsohn C, Kastner P, Krust A, Garnier JM, Ruffenach F, Leroy P and Chambon P: Differentially expressed isoforms of the mouse retinoic acid receptor ß are generated by usage of two promoters and alternative splicing. EMBO J 1991 (10):71-81

128 Nagpal S, Zelent A and Chambon P: RAR-ß4, a retinoic acid receptor isoform, is generated from RAR-ß2 by alternative splicing and usage of a CUG initiator codon. Proc Natl Acad Sci USA 1992 (89):2718-2722

129 Leid M, Kastner P and Chambon P: Multiplicity generates diversity in the retinoic acid signalling pathways. Trends Biochem Sci 1992 (17):427-433
130 Ruberte E, Kastner P, Dolle P, Krust A, Leroy P, Mendelsohn C, Zelent A and Chambon P: Retinoic acid receptors in the embryo. Dev Biol 1991 (2):153-159
131 Brand NJ, Petkovich M and Chambon P: Characterization of a functional promoter for the human retinoic acid receptor-alpha (hRAR-α). Nucleic Acids Res 1990 (18):6799-6806
132 Leroy A, Nakshatri H and Chambon P: Mouse retinoic acid receptor-α2 isoform is transcribed from a promoter that contains a retinoic acid response element. Proc Natl Acad Sci USA 1991 (88):10138-10142
133 Wang L-H, Tsai SY, Cook RG, Beattie WG, Tsai M-J and O'Malley BW: COUP transcription factor is a member of the steroid receptor superfamily. Nature 1989 (340):163-166
134 Oro AE, McKeown M and Evans RM: Relationship between the product of the *Drosophila ultraspiracle* locus and the vertebrate retinoid X receptor. Nature 1990 (347):298-301
135 Mangelsdorf DJ, Ong ES, Dyck JA and Evans RM: Nuclear receptor that identifies a novel retinoic acid response pathway. Nature 1990 (345):224-229
136 Leid M, Kastner P, Lyons R, Nakshatri H, Saunders M, Zacharewski T, Chen J-Y, Staub A, Garnier J-M, Mader S and Chambon P: Purification, cloning, and RXR identity of the HeLa cell factor with which RAR or TR heterodimerizes to bind target sequences efficiently. Cell 1992 (68):377-395
137 Mangelsdorf DJ, Borgmeyer U, Heyman RA, Zhou JY, Ong ES, Oro AE, Kakizuka A and Evans RM: Characterization of three RXR genes that mediate the action of 9-*cis* retinoic acid. Genes Dev 1992 (6):329-344
138 Fleischhauer K, Park JH, DiSanto JP, Marks M, Ozato K and Yang SY: Isolation of a full-length cDNA clone encoding a N-terminally variant form of the human retinoid X receptor ß. Nucleic Acids Res 1992 (20):1801
139 Liu Q and Linney E: The mouse retinoid-X receptor-γ gene: genomic organization and evidence for functional isoforms. Mol Endocrinol 1993 (7):651-658
140 Glass CK, Devary OV and Rosenfeld MG: Multiple cell type-specific proteins differentially regulate target sequence recognition by the α retinoic acid receptor. Cell 1990 (63):729-738
141 Yu V, Naar AM and Rosenfeld MG: Transcriptional regulation by the nuclear receptor superfamily. Current Opinion in Biotechnology 1992 (3):597-602
142 Yu VC, Delsert C, Andersen B, Holloway JM, Devary OV, Naar AM, Kim SY, Boutin J-M, Glass CK and Rosenfeld MG: RXRß: a coregulator that enhances binding of retinoic acid, thyroid hormone, and vitamin D receptors to their cognate response elements. Cell 1991 (67):1251-1266
143 Kliewer SA, Umesono K, Mangelsdorf DJ and Evans RM: Retinoid X receptor interacts with nuclear receptors in retinoic acid, thyroid hormone and vitamin D3 signalling. Nature 1992 (355):446-449
144 Kliewer SA, Umesono K, Noonan DJ, Heyman RA and Evans RM: Convergence of 9-*cis* retinoic acid and peroxisome proliferator signalling pathways through heterodimer formation of their receptors. Nature 1992 (358):771-774
145 Kliewer SA, Umesono K, Heyman RA, Mangelsdorf DJ, Dyck JA and Evans RM: Retinoid X receptor-COUP-TF interactions modulate retinoic acid signaling. Proc Natl Acad Sci USA 1992 (89):1448-1452
146 Thomas HE, Stunnenberg HG and Stewart AF: Heterodimerization of the *Drosophila* ecdysone receptor with retinoid X receptor and *ultraspiracle*. Nature 1993 (362):471-475
147 Green S: Promiscuous liaisons. Nature 1993 (361):590-591
148 Heyman RA, Mangelsdorf DJ, Dyck JA, Stein RB, Eichele G, Evans RM and Thaller C: 9-cis retinoic acid is a high affinity ligand for the retinoid X receptor. Cell 1992 (68):397-406
149 Levin AA, Sturzenbecker LJ, Kazmer S, Bosakowski T, Huselton C, Allenby G, Speck J, Kratzeisen C, Rosenberger M, Lovey A and Grippo JF: 9-*cis* retinoic acid stereoisomer binds and activates the nuclear receptor RXR-α. Nature 1992 (355):359-361
150 Zhang X-k, Lehmann J, Hoffmann B, Dawson MI, Cameron J, Graupner G, Hermann T, Tran P and Pfahl M: Homodimer formation of retinoid X receptor induced by 9-*cis* retinoic acid. Nature 1992 (358):587-591
151 Damm K, Thompson CC and Evans RM: Protein encoded by v-*erb*A functions as a thyroid-hormone receptor antagonist. Nature 1989 (339):593-597
152 Sap J, Munoz A, Schmitt J, Stunnenberg H and Vennstrom B: Repression of transcription mediated at a thyroid hormone response element by the v-erb-A oncogene product. Nature 1989 (340):242-244
153 Saatcioglu F, Deng T and Karin M: A novel cis element mediating ligand-independent activation by c-ErbA: implications for hormonal regulation. Cell 1993 (75):1095-1105
154 Lehmann JM, Zhang X-K, Graupner G, Lee M-O, Hermann T, Hoffmann B and Pfahl M: Formation of retinoid X receptor homodimers leads to repression of T_3 response: hormonal cross talk by ligand-induced squelching. Mol Cell Biol 1993 (13):7698-7707
155 Barettino D, Bugge TH, Bartunek P, del Mar Vivanco-Ruiz M, Sonntag-Buck V, Beug H, Zenke M and Stunnenberg HG: Unliganded T_3R, but not its oncogenic variant, v-erbA, suppresses RAR-dependent transactivation by titrating out RXR. EMBO J 1993 (12):1343-1354
156 Green S and Chambon P: Oestradiol induction of a glucocorticoid-responsive gene by a chimaeric receptor. Nature 1987 (325):75-78
157 Mader S, Kumar V, de Verneuil H and Chambon P: Three amino acids of the oestrogen receptor are essential to its ability to distinguish an oestrogen

from a glucocorticoid-responsive element. Nature 1989 (338):271-274
158 Umesono K and Evans RM: Determinants of target gene specificity for steroid/tyroid hormone receptors. Cell 1989 (57):1139-1146
159 Umesono K, Giguere V, Glass CK, Rosenfeld MG and Evans RM: Retinoic acid and thyroid hormone induce gene expression through a common responsive element. Nature 1988 (336):262-265
160 de The H, del Mar Vivanco-Ruiz M, Tiollais P, Stunnenberg H and Dejean A: Identification of a retinoic acid responsive element in the retinoic acid receptor ß gene. Nature 1990 (343):177-180
161 Sucov HM, Murakami KK and Evans RM: Characterization of an autoregulated response element in the mouse retinoic acid receptor type ß gene. Proc Natl Acad Sci USA 1990 (87):5392-5396
162 Lehmann JM, Zhang X-K and Pfahl M: RARγ2 expression is regulated through a retinoic acid response element embedded in sp1 sites. Mol Cell Biol 1992 (12):2976-2985
163 Munoz-Canoves P, Vik DP and Tack BF: Mapping of a retinoic acid-responsive element in the promoter region of the complement factor H gene. J Biol Chem 1990 (265):20065-20068
164 Popperl H and Featherstone MS: Identification of a retinoic acid response element upstream of the murine *Hox-4.2* gene. Mol Cell Biol 1993 (13):257-265
165 Widom RL, Ladias JAA, Kouidou S and Karathanasis SK: Synergistic interactions between transcription factors control expression of the apolipoprotein AI gene in liver cells. Mol Cell Biol 1991 (11):677-687
166 Naar AM, Boutin J-M, Lipkin SM, Yu VC, Holloway JM, Glass CK and Rosenfeld MG: The orientation and spacing of core DNA-binding motifs dictate selective transcriptional responses to three nuclear receptors. Cell 1991 (65):1267-1279
167 Umesono K, Murakami KK, Thompson CC and Evans RM: Direct repeats as selective response elements for the thyroid hormone, retinoic acid, and vitamin D3 receptors. Cell 1991 (65):1255-1266
168 Carlberg C, Bendik I, Wyss A, Meier E, Sturzenbecker LJ, Grippo JF and Hunziker W: Two nuclear signalling pathways for vitamin D. Nature 1993 (361):657-660
169 Tini M, Otulakowski G, Breitman ML, Tsui L-C and Giguere V: An everted repeat mediates retinoic acid induction of the γF-cyrstallin gene: evidence of a direct role for retinoids in lens development. Genes Dev 1993 (7):295-307
170 Durand B, Saunders M, Leroy P, Leid M and Chambon P: All-*trans* and 9-*cis* retinoic acid induction of CRABPII transcription is mediated by RAR-RXR heterodimers bound to DR1 and DR2 repeated motifs. Cell 1992 (71):73-85
171 Smith WC, Nakshatri H, Leroy P, Rees J and Chambon P: A retinoic acid response element is present in the mouse cellular retinol binding protein I (mCRBPI) promoter. EMBO J 1991 (10):2223-2230
172 Mader S, Chen J-Y, Chen Z, White J, Chambon P and Gronemeyer H: The patterns of binding of RAR, RXR and TR homo- and heterodimers to direct repeats are dictated by the binding specificities of the DNA binding domains. EMBO J 1993 (12):5029-5041
173 Nagpal S, Saunders M, Kastner P, Durand B, Nakshatri H and Chambon P: Promoter context- and response element-dependent specificity of the transcriptional activation and modulating functions of retinoic acid receptors. Cell 1992 (70):1007-1019
174 Nagpal S, Friant S, Nakshatri H and Chambon P: RARs and RXRs: evidence for two autonomous transactivation functions (AF-1 and AF-2) and heterodimerization *in vivo*. EMBO J 1993 (12):2349-2360
175 Perlmann T, Rangarajan PN, Umesono K and Evans RM: Determinants for selective RAR and TR recognition of direct repeat HREs. Genes Dev 1993 (7):1411-1422
176 Wilson TE, Paulsen RE, Padgett KA and Milbrandt J: Participation of non-zinc finger residues in DNA binding by two nuclear orphan receptors. Science 1992 (256):107-110
177 Towers TL, Luisi BF, Asianov A and Freedman LP: DNA target selectivity by the vitamin D3 receptor: mechanism of dimer binding to an asymmetric repeat element. Proc Natl Acad Sci USA 1993 (90):6310-6314
178 Kurokawa R, Yu VC, Naar A, Kyakumoto S, Han Z, Silverman S, Rosenfeld MG and Glass CK: Differential orientations of the DNA-binding domain and carboxy-terminal dimerization interface regulate binding site selection by nuclear receptor heterodimers. Genes Dev 1993 (7):1423-1435
179 Abate C and Curran T: Encounters with Fos and Jun on the road to AP-1. Semin Cancer Biol 1990 (1):19-26
180 Hai T and Curran T: Cross-family dimerization of transcription factors Fos/Jun and ATF/CREB alters DNA binding specificity. Proc Natl Acad Sci USA 1991 (88):3720-3724
181 Benezra R, Davis RL, Lockshon D, Turner DL and Weintraub H: The protein id: a negative regulator of helix-loop-helix DNA binding proteins. Cell 1990 (61):49-59
182 Lassar AB, Davis RL, Wright WE, Kadesch T, Murre C, Voronova A, Baltimore D and Weintraub H: Functional activity of myogenic HLH proteins requires hetero-oligomerization with E12/E47-like proteins in vivo. Cell 1991 (66):305-315
183 Ruberte E, Dolle P, Chambon P and Morriss-Kay G: Retinoic acid receptors and cellular retinoid binding proteins II. Their differential pattern of transcription during early morphogenesis in mouse embryos. Development 1991 (111):45-60
184 Dolle P, Ruberte E, Leroy P, Morriss-Kay G and Chambon P: Retinoic acid receptors and cellular retinoid binding proteins I. A systematic study of their differential pattern of transcription during mouse organogenesis. Development 1990 (110):1133-1151
185 Rowe A, Eager NSC and Brickell PM: A member of the RXR nuclear receptor family is expressed in

neural-crest-derived cells of the developing chick peripheral nervous system. Development 1991 (111):771-778
186 Lufkin T, Lohnes D, Mark M, Dierich A, Gorry P, Gaub M-P, LeMeur M and Chambon P: High postnatal lethality and testis degeneration in retinoic acid receptor α mutant mice. Proc Natl Acad Sci USA 1993 (90):7225-7229
187 Li E, Sucov HM, Lee K-F, Evans RM and Jaenisch R: Normal development and growth of mice carrying a targeted disruption of the α1 retinoic acid receptor gene. Proc Natl Acad Sci USA 1993 (90):1590-1594
188 Lohnes D, Kastner P, Dierich A, Mark M, LeMeur M and Chambon P: Function of retinoic acid receptor γ in the mouse. Cell 1993 (73):643-658
189 Tautz D: Redundancies, development and the flow of information. BioEssays 1992 (14):263-266
190 Weintraub H: The MyoD family and myogenesis: redundancy, networks, and thresholds. Cell 1993 (75):1241-1244
191 Lafyatis R, Kim S-J, Angel P, Roberts AB, Sporn MB, Karin M and Wilder RL: Interleukin-1 stimulates and all-*trans*-retinoic acid inhibits collagenase gene expression through its 5' activator protein-1-binding site. Mol Endocrinol 1990 (4):973-980
192 Schule R, Rangarajan P, Yang N, Kliewer S, Ransone LJ, Bolado J, Verma IM and Evans RM: Retinoic acid is a negative regulator of AP-1 responsive genes. Proc Natl Acad Sci USA 1991 (88):6092-6096
193 Yang-Yen H-F, Zhang X-k, Graupner G, Tzukerman M, Sakamoto B, Karin M and Pfahl M: Antagonism between retinoic acid receptors and AP-1: implications for tumor promotion and inflammation. The New Biologist 1991 (3):1206-1219
194 Gaub MP, Rochette-Egly C, Lutz Y, Ali S, Matthes H, Scheuer I and Chambon P: Immunodetection of multiple species of retinoic acid receptor α: evidence for phosphorylation. Exp Cell Res 1992 (201):335-346
195 Rochette-Egly C, Gaub M-P, Lutz Y, Ali S, Scheuer I and Chambon P: Retinoic acid receptor-β: immunodetection and phosphorylation on tyrosine residues. Mol Endocrinol 1992 (6):2197-2209
196 Rochette-Egly C, Lutz Y, Saunders M, Scheuer I, Gaub M-P and Chambon P: Retinoic acid receptor γ: specific immunodetection and phosphorylation. J Cell Biol 1991 (115):535-545
197 Huggenvik JI, Collard MW, Kim Y-W and Sharma RP: Modification of the retinoic acid signaling pathway by the catalytic subunit of protein kinase-A. Mol Endocrinol 1993 (7):543-550
198 Power RF, Mani SK, Codina J, Conneelly OM and O'Malley BW: Dopaminergic and ligand-independent activation of steroid hormone receptors. Science 1991 (254):1636-1639
199 Bishop JM: Oncogenes as hormone receptors. Nature 1986 (321):112-113
200 Green S and Chambon P: A superfamily of potentially oncogenic hormone receptors. Nature 1986 (324):615-617
201 Zenke M, Munoz A, Sap J, Vennstrom B and Beug H: v-*erb*A oncogene activation entails the loss of hormone-dependent regulator activity of c-*erb*A. Cell 1990 (61):1035-1049
202 Sharif M and Privalsky ML: v-*erbA* oncogene function in neoplasia correlates with its ability to repress retinoic acid receptor action. Cell 1991 (66):885-893
203 Desbois C, Aubert D, Legrand C, Pain B and Samarut J: A novel mechanism of action for v-ErbA: abrogation of the inactivation of transcription factor AP-1 by retinoic acid and thyroid hormone receptors. Cell 1991 (67):731-740
204 Warrell RP, de Thé H, Wang Z-Y and Degos L: Acute promyelocytic leukemia. N Engl J Med 1993 (329):177-189
205 Grignani F, Fagioli M, Alcalay M, Longo L, Pandolfi PP, Donti E, Biondi A, Lo Coco F, Grignani F and Pelicci PG: Acute promyelocytic leukemia: from genetics to treatment. Blood 1994 (83):10-25
206 Zelent A: Translocation of the RARα locus to the PML or PLZF gene in acute promyelocytic leukaemia. Br J Haematol 1994 (86):451-460
207 Houle B, Rochette-Egly C and Bradley WEC: Tumor-suppressive effect of the retinoic acid receptor β in human epidermoid lung cancer cells. Proc Natl Acad Sci USA 1993 (90):985-989
208 Gebert JF, Moghal N, Frangioni JV, Sugarbaker DJ and Neel BG: High frequency of retinoic acid receptor β abnormalities in human lung cancer. Oncogene 1991 (16):1859-1868
209 de Thé H, Marchio A, Tiollais P and Dejean A: A novel steroid thyroid hormone receptor-related gene inappropriately expressed in human hepatocellular carcinoma. Nature 1987 (330):667-670
210 Garcia M, de Thé H, Tiollais P, Samarut J and Dejean A: A hepatitis B virus pre-S-retinoic acid receptor β chimera transforms erythrocytic progenitor cells *in vitro*. Proc Natl Acad Sci USA 1993 (90):89-93
211 Takahashi N and Breitman TR: Covalent modification of proteins by ligands of steroid hormone receptors. Proc Natl Acad Sci USA 1992 (89):10807-10811
212 Buck J, Derguini F, Levi E, Nakanishi K and Hammerling U: Intracellular signaling by 14-hydroxy-4,14-*retro*-retinol. Science 1991 (254):1654-1656
213 Leroy P, Krust A, Zelent A, Mendelsohn C, Garnier J-M, Kastner P, Dierich A and Chambon P: Multiple isoforms of the mouse retinoic acid receptor-α are generated by alternative splicing and differential induction by retinoic acid. EMBO J 1991 (10):59-69
214 van der Leede B-J, Folkers GE, Kruyt FAE and van der Saag PT: Genomic organization of the human retinoic acid receptor β2. Biochem Biophys Res Commun 1992 (188):695-702
215 Kastner P, Krust A, Mendelsohn C, Garnier JM, Zelent A, Leroy P, Staub A and Chambon P: Murine isoforms of retinoic acid receptor γ with specific patterns of expression. Proc Natl Acad Sci USA 1990 (87):2700-2704

216 Lehmann JM, Hoffmann B and Pfahl M: Genomic organization of the retinoic acid receptor gamma gene. Nucleic Acids Res 1991 (19):573-578
217 Hughes MR, Malloy PJ, Kieback DG, Kesterson RA, Pike JW, Feldman D and O'Malley BW: Point mutations in the human vitamin D receptor gene associated with hypocalcemic rickets. Science 1988 (242):1702-1705

Cellular Biology of the Retinoids

Reuben Lotan

Department of Tumor Biology, University of Texas M.D. Anderson Cancer Center, Houston, Texas 77030, U.S.A.

Although interest in cellular biology of vitamin A metabolites and synthetic analogues, collectively called retinoids, has been increasing steadily over the last 15 years, it has seen a very sharp rise during the last few years. A review published in 1980 [1] contained less than 400 references, whereas a recent literature search indicated that nearly 5000 papers, many reviews [e.g. 2-6], and books [e.g. 7-10] have been published between 1988 and 1994 on retinoids. Retinoids have attracted the attention and research efforts of embryologists, developmental biologists, cell biologists, molecular biologists, dermatologists, and investigators interested in cancer prevention and therapy because they modulate the growth and differentiation of normal, premalignant, and malignant epithelial and mesenchymal cells *in vitro* and *in vivo*. Naturally occurring retinoids act as physiologic regulators of embryonal development and maintain the proper differentiation of many tissues in the adult. Retinoids also act pharmacologically to restore regulation of differentiation and growth in certain premalignant and malignant cells *in vitro* and *in vivo*.

The encouraging results of a few clinical trials of prevention and therapy have stimulated the efforts to further elucidate the mechanism of retinoid action at the cellular and molecular levels. This review highlights some of the pleiotropic cellular and biochemical effects of retinoids on cancer cells (Table 1) and considers their clinical implications. Emphasis is placed here on cells derived from solid tumours as other chapters deal with effects of retinoids on haematological malignancies. References will be limited to reviews and recent publications through which readers interested in additional information can reach earlier original publications.

Effects of Retinoids on Anchorage-Dependent and Anchorage-Independent Growth

The growth and differentiation of various normal and malignant cells in culture is modulated (stimulated or inhibited) by retinoids [11]. Most of the cultured malignant cells exhibit inhibition of anchorage-dependent growth and anchorage-independent growth [1,11,12]. The growth of a few cell lines was found to be stimulated by retinoids [13]. The most frequently observed effect of retinoids on tumour cells *in vitro* is inhibition of anchorage-dependent growth. Many tumour cell types including melanoma, neuroblastoma, glioma, retinoblastoma, embryonal carcinoma, carcinomas of the lung, breast, prostate, bladder, colon, skin, head and neck, cervix, and various types of sarcoma that grow as adherent monolayers on plastic tissue culture dishes often exhibit a decrease in growth rate and saturation density after exposure to retinoids [11]. These effects occur in the retinoid concentration range between 1 nM and 10 μM and are dependent on the dose and duration of treatment (Fig. 1). DNA synthesis is suppressed within 12 to 24 hours of treatment initiation, the cells are either arrested or accumulate in G_1 phase of the cell cycle or in S phase of the cell cycle and growth inhibition can be detected within 24 to 72 hours, depending on the doubling time of the cells. In some cells (e.g., a subline of human MCF-7 breast carcinoma) growth stimulation was observed at low RA concentrations (1 nM and 10 nM) whereas growth inhibition was evident at higher concentrations (0.1 and 1 μM) [14]. The number of cell colonies on plastic tissue culture dishes and their size decreases after retinoid treatment

Table 1. Pleiotropic cellular and biochemical effects of retinoids*

Cell growth and viability

1. Inhibition of cell growth (changes in growth factors and growth factor receptors)
2. Stimulation of cell growth
3. Inhibition of colony formation in semi-solid medium
4. Cytotoxicity
5. Induction of apoptosis (tissue transglutaminase; *Bcl*-2; TGF-ß)

Cell differentiation

1. Stimulation of differentiation (see Table 2)
2. Inhibition of differentiation (see Table 2)

Cellular interactions

1. Cell-cell communication (connexin 43)
2. Cell-cell and cell extracellular matrix adhesion (desmosomes; integrins, laminin, fibronectin, proteoglycans, hyaluronic acid)

Cell surface

1. *De novo* expression of antigens (ICAM-1; NCAM, SSEA-1; MHC class I)
2. Altered structure of membrane glycoproteins (glycosylation)
3. Altered lipids and glycolipids (GD2; acylceramide; fatty acids)

Signal transduction

1. Expression of cell surface receptors for cytokines [EGF-R; HER2/*neu*; PDGF-R; NGF-R; TrkB; HGF-R (c-met); IL-2-R; IL-6-R]
2. Function of receptors (protein kinase activity)
3. Expression of cytokines/growth factors (TGF-α; TGF-ß; Hst-1/kFGF; PDGF; MK; IGF-I; IGF-II; IL-1; IL-2; IL-3; IL-6)
4. Induction of membrane channels (glutamate receptor channels)
5. Modulation of signalling pathways and second messengers (pKA; pKC; cyclic AMP; IP4; 2'-5'-adenylate synthetase)

Oncogene expression

1. Suppression of oncogene expression (c-*myc*, N-*myc*; c-*myb*, c-*mos*)
2. Induction of proto-oncogene expression (*erb*-B1; c-*fos*; c-*jun*; c-*kit*; c-*raf*; c-*src*)

Cell cycle regulatory components

1. Induction of RB gene or suppression of RB protein phosphorylation
2. Suppression of p34 cdc kinase

Regulation of gene expression

1. Direct effect by binding of nuclear RA receptors to RARE or RXRE in gene promoter region (RAR-ß; laminin; Homeobox genes; alcohol dehydrogenase
2. Indirect regulation via induction of transcription factors (c-*jun*; AP-2; Egr-1)
3. Antagonism of gene activation by binding of nuclear RA receptors to other transcription factors e.g. *jun-fos* (stromelysin; collagenase)

*Examples of molecules that may be involved in the effects are given in parentheses
TGF, transforming growth factor; CAM, cell adhesion molecule; MHC, major histocompatibility complex; EGF, epidermal growth factor; PDGF, platelet-derived growth factor; NGF, nerve growth factor; TrkB, neurotrophin receptor; HGF, hepatocyte growth factor; IL, interleukin; FGF, fibroblast growth factor; MK, midkine; IGF, insulin-like growth factor; pKA, cyclic adenosine monophosphate-dependent protein kinase; pKC, protein kinase type C; RB, retinoblastoma; RARE, RA response element

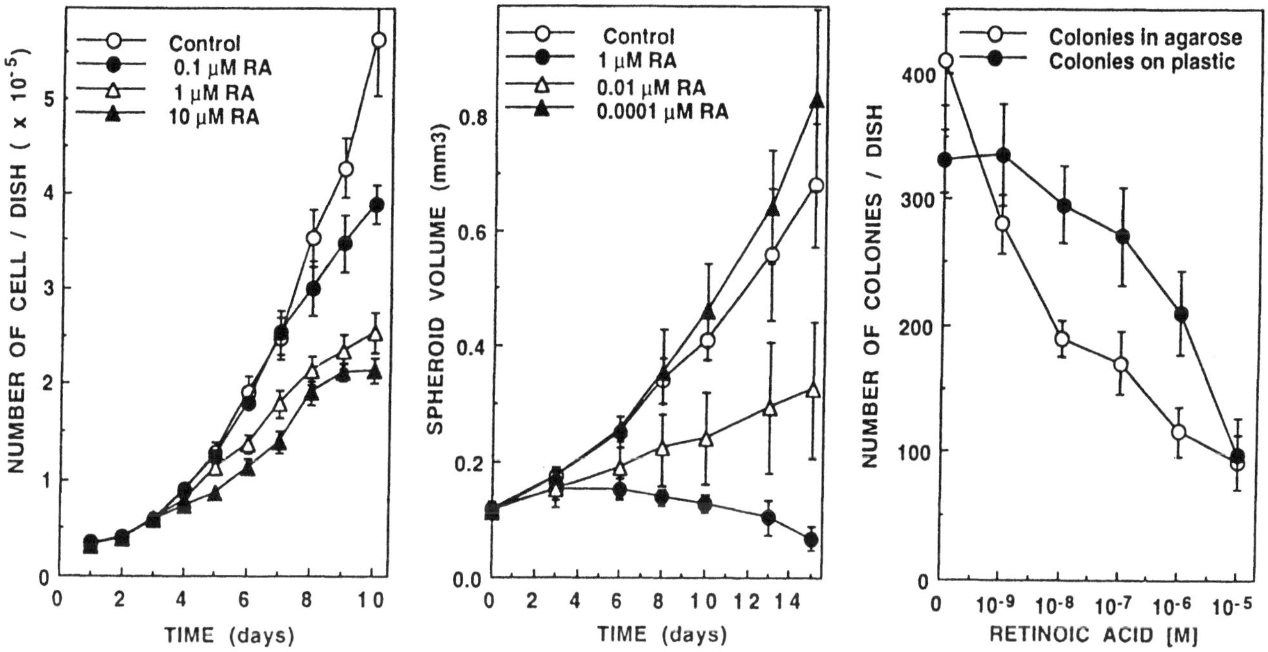

Fig. 1. ß-All-*trans* retinoic acid (RA) dose-dependent and time-dependent inhibition of human head and neck squamous carcinoma cell (HNSCC) proliferation, multicellular spheroid growth, and colony formation. (Left panel) Cells (line 1483) were seeded in tissue culture dishes and after 24 h, and at 72-h intervals thereafter, the cultures were fed control medium or one containing the indicated RA concentrations. At the indicated times, the cells were detached and counted. The results are presented as the mean ± SE of triplicate cultures. (Middle panel) Inhibition of the growth of human HNSCC multicellular spheroids. Spheroids of similar diameter were placed individually in each well of a 24-multiwell plate that had been precoated with 1.25% agarose and fed control medium or one supplemented with the indicated RA concentrations. After 72 h, and at 72-h intervals thereafter, the spheroids received fresh medium without or with RA. At the indicated times 2 perpendicular diameters of the spheroids were measured using an inverted microscope with a calibrated reticle and their volume was calculated. The values represent the mean ± SE of 6 spheroids. (Right panel) Inhibition of 1483 HNSCC colony formation on plastic or in agarose. Colony formation on plastic was analysed using a microscope after cells were treated with RA every 72 h for 14 days. The effect of RA on colony formation in semisolid agarose was determined using an inverted microscope after treatment with RA every 72 h for 14 days. The results are presented as the mean ± SE of triplicate dishes.

(Fig. 1). Maintenance of the growth-inhibited state usually requires the continuous presence of retinoids as their removal from the culture medium often results in a reversal of the growth inhibitory effects within 24 to 72 hours. The growth of several types of cell, in particular many haematopoietic cells such as lymphomas, leukaemias, myelomas, premonocytic leukaemia, promyelocytic leukaemia that normally grow in suspension can be inhibited by retinoids. Some solid tumour cells can grow as tightly packed multicellular spheroids suspended in liquid medium. The growth of such spheroids is also suppressed by retinoids [12]. Many tumour cells exhibit an anchorage-independent growth as colonies in agar, agarose or methyl cellulose, and this growth is considered to be a hallmark of malignant transformation as it distinguishes malignant from normal cells. Treatment of various transformed and tumour cells with retinoids restores anchorage dependence and inhibits the ability of the cells to grow in suspension (Fig. 1). The effective concentrations of retinoids for inhibition of tumour cell growth in culture are often pharmacological and not physiological. However, quite a large number of tumour cells are inhibited considerably even at physiological doses (1 µM for retinol and 0.01 µM for RA). Often cells that are only marginally inhibited in monolayer culture show marked inhibition of anchorage-independent growth in agarose, suggesting that the inhibition of anchorage-independent growth is a more sensitive assay for the suppression of the growth of tumour cells by retinoids [11,12,15]. This assay has also been performed with cells dissociated from fresh tumour biopsies and has demonstrated sensitivity of different tumour cells to different retinoids [16-18].

Cytotoxicity of Retinoids and their Effect on Apoptosis

In addition to the cytostatic effects of retinoids discussed above, these compounds have also been shown to exert non-specific cytotoxic effects and to induce programmed cell death. At concentrations higher than 50 μM, many retinoids exhibit cytotoxic effects on most cells. This toxicity of retinoids is probably due to their detergent-like effects at high concentrations. The cytotoxicity is enhanced in serum-free medium, possibly because of the absence of serum albumin, which binds retinoids.

Retinoids also induce programmed cell death (apoptosis) in mesenchymal, neuro-ectodermal, haematopoietic and epithelial cells during normal development and in cultured untransformed and tumour cells. The effects of retinoids are often associated with the induction of tissue transglutaminase (tTG), DNA fragmentation indicative of endogenous endonuclease activation, and nuclear condensation [19-21]. RA treatment of human cervical carcinoma HeLa-TV or neuroblastoma SK-N-BE resulted in a 6 to 12-fold increase in tTG and a parallel increase in the apoptotic index. The spontaneous apoptosis in cultured clones of the neuroblastoma SK-N-BE cells occurred only in undifferentiated cells and was not observed in cells showing neurite outgrowth (N-type). Such cells have been found to express p26-*Bcl*-2 oncoprotein, which is known to block apoptosis. Interestingly, RA treatment that induced neuronal differentiation in SK-N-BE clones also increased the level of p26-*Bcl*-2. These results indicate that RA-induced apoptosis was independent of the neuronal differentiation induced by RA in the neuroblastoma cultures [19]. In contrast, RA enhanced apoptosis in HL-60 myeloid leukaemia cells after 6-8 days subsequent to inducing cell differentiation into neutrophil-like cells [22]. A possible explanation for this observation and the similar finding of differentiation *in vitro* of acute promyelocytic leukaemia cells by RA is suppression of the level of p26-*Bcl*-2 protein in the differentiated leukaemia cells [23]. Yet another pattern of apoptosis induction that is independent of differentiation has been observed recently in several human lymphoma and leukaemia cells treated with the synthetic retinoid N-(4-hydroxyphenyl)retinamide (HPR) [24]. HPR caused cytostatic effects at concentrations of 0.3 and 1 μM, whereas apoptosis was induced at concentrations of 3 μM or higher [24]. The characteristic fragmentation of DNA was observed after 24 hours of treatment, however, the more sensitive method of intracellular labelling of DNA breaks with fluorescent dUTP was able to detect apoptotic cells as early as 6 hours after HPR treatment initiation. This rapid effect was specific to HPR as all-*trans* retinoic acid only caused apoptosis at later times subsequent to inducing cell differentiation [22-24]. Interestingly, HPR induced apoptosis in RA-resistant mutant HL-60 leukaemia cells suggesting a distinct mechanism of action that is independent of the known nuclear retinoic acid receptors, which do not bind HPR and are not transactivated by this retinoid [24].

Although the mechanism of apoptosis induction by retinoids is still not fully understood, the likely mediators of this effect are the enzyme tTG that is often associated with apoptosis and suppression of *Bcl*-2 expression following differentiation [20-23]. However, as mentioned above, other mechanisms are implicated in the effects of HPR [24]. Indirect effects of retinoids on cell death may also be mediated via induction of transforming growth factor-ß, which has been found to increase in cells undergoing apoptosis [25].

Effects of Retinoids on Cell Differentiation

The physiological functions of naturally occurring retinoids include regulation of embryonal development and maintenance of the proper differentiation of many epithelial and mesenchymal tissues in the adult [8]. Retinoids also act pharmacologically to restore regulation of differentiation in certain malignant cells *in vitro* (Fig. 2 and Table 2). The effects of retinoids on cell differentiation have been studied extensively in a few defined systems primarily in cultured cell lines derived from embryonal carcinoma (EC), normal and malignant keratinocytes, premonocytic and myeloid leukaemias, neuroblastoma, and melanoma. In most of

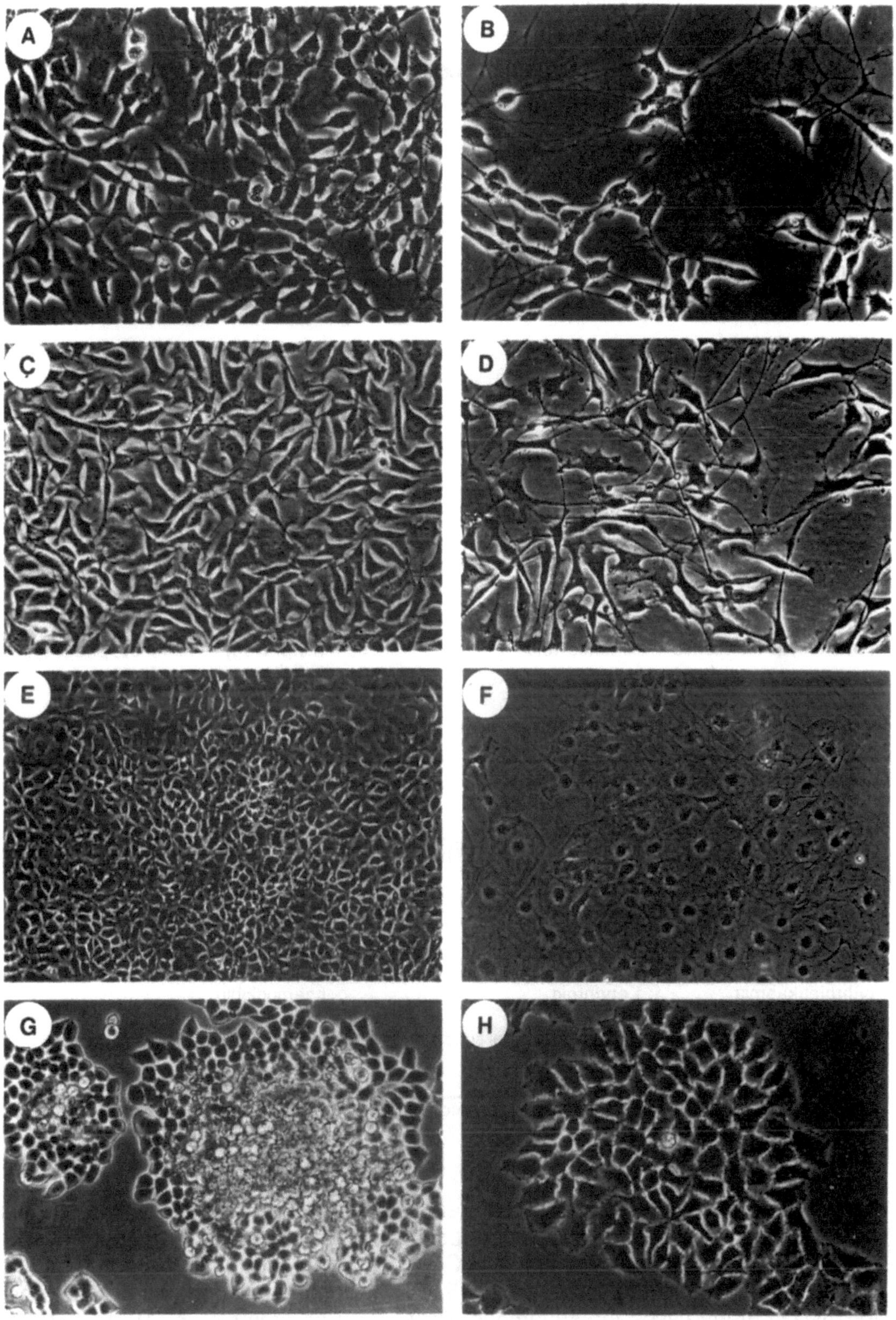

Fig. 2. Photomicrographs of tumour cells grown in the absence (A, C, E and G) or presence (B, D, F and H) of 1 μM RA for 7 days. (A, B) Human SK-N-SH neuroblastoma cells. (C, D) Mouse K-1735 melanoma cells. (E, F) Human PA-1 teratocarcinoma cells. (G, H) Human HeLa-S3 cervical carcinoma cells. The cells were photographed using a phase contrast Nikon microscope

Table 2. Retinoids and differentiation of human tumor cells *in vitro*

Tumour type	Differentiation induced	Markers analysed
Embryonal carcinoma	neuronal	morphology, homeobox genes; SSEA-3 suppression; neurofilament; glutamate-R channels
Non seminomatous germ cell tumour	ectodermal mesodermal endodermal	keratin; GFAP; neurofilaments, extracellular matrix
Choriocarcinoma	syncytio-trophoblastic	human chorionic gonadotrophin
Neuroblastoma	neuronal	morphology, enolase; calcyclin; NGF-R calcium channels
Astrocytoma	astrocytic	GFAP
Medulloblastoma	astrocytic	
Retinoblastoma	photoreceptor	Flexner-Winter-Steiner rosettes
Melanoma	melanocytic	morphology, melanin; tyrosinase
Myeloid leukaemia	myeloid	morphology; NBT reduction surface antigens
Premonocytic leukaemia	monocytoid	morphology, adherence; phagocytic leukaemia activity, surface antigens
Rhabdomyosarcoma	myogenic	myotubes; creatine kinase
Colon carcinoma		CEA
Breast carcinoma	mammary	casein, lipids
Small cell lung carcinoma	squamous differentiation suppressed	keratin; involucrin desmosomes
Variant small cell lung carcinoma	classic	morphology
Erythroleukaemia	erythroid	haemoglobin
Squamous carcinoma	Squamous differentiation suppressed	keratin K1, involucrin; TGase I

SSEA, stage-specific embryonic antigen; R, receptor; GFAP, glial fibrillar acidic protein; NBT, nitroblue tetrazolium; CEA, carcinoembryonic antigen

these cell types, retinoids enhance differentiation (Table 2). However, in cultured keratinocytes and squamous cell carcinomas (SCCs), retinoids inhibit squamous differentiation [5,26]. Because in many cases the squamous differentiation of normally nonkeratinising epithelial cells is aberrant, the effect of retinoids can be viewed as restoration of the normal non-keratinising phenotype [26].

The ability of retinoids to induce distinct pathways of differentiation indicates that they do not determine the direction of differentiation but rather enhance predetermined programmes in cells that have the potential to undergo differentiation along one or more specific pathways. For example, in F9 EC cells, retinoids induce endodermal differentiation [27] whereas in human embryonal carcinoma cells retinoids induce a neuronal differentiation [28]. In P19 EC cells retinoids can induce both myogenic differentiation and neuronal differentiation depending on the concentration of retinoid used [29]. In HL-60 myeloid leukaemia cells that have the potential to undergo either myeloid or monocytoid differentiation, retinoids can only induce the myeloid pathway [30]. In contrast, RA was able to induce 3 different pathways, ectodermal, mesodermal, and endodermal in a developmentally pluripotent germ cell tumour [31]. Thus, the effect of retinoids on the differentiation pathway appears to depend on other cellular factors that are either expressed in the cells constitutively (e.g. certain transcription factors), or are induced by retinoic acid and then turn on a specific differentiation pathway (e.g. Hox genes [32]; AP-2 [33]).

Because of their ability to enhance the differentiation of malignant cells, retinoids have been frontrunners in "differentiation therapy" trials aimed at inducing the differentiation of tumour cells *in vivo* [6]. Some of the concepts underlying this approach are also applicable to chemoprevention. For example, agents that can reverse the aberrant differentiation state of preneoplastic cells to a normal state may prevent carcinogenesis by suppressing the growth of the cells as a result of restoration of responses to normal growth controlling mechanisms. Retinoid-induced differentiation of teratocarcinoma cells prevented gene amplification [34]. If retinoids can exert a similar effect on premalignant cells, then their conversion to malignant cells via events requiring gene amplification could be suppressed.

The induction of differentiation of tumour cells was not restricted to established cell lines since fresh leukaemic cells in short-term culture were also responsive to retinoid treatment [35; see also the chapter by de Thé et al. in this volume]. A major development in the clinical application of retinoids was the discovery that all-*trans* RA can induce the differentiation of acute promyelocytic leukaemia cells *in vivo.* Another application of the ability of RA to induce differentiation *in vitro* of fresh leukaemic cells has been proposed for purging leukaemic cells in murine bone marrow expansion cultures [36]. There are only limited reports regarding induction of differentiation of solid tumour cells *in vivo* and they are restricted to murine embryonal carcinoma cells injected into syngeneic mice. A significant degree of differentiation was observed in teratocarcinomas when RA was injected directly into the tumour [37] or when several retinoids were administered in the diet [38].

Several clinically relevant concepts have emerged from recent studies on the effect of retinoid-induced differentiation on response of tumour cells to cytotoxic agents. It has been found that RA-induced differentiation of murine PCC4 EC cells increased severalfold their sensitivity to cisplatin (CDDP) and VP16 *in vitro* and the combination of RA and CDDP was also more effective in reducing tumour growth *in vivo* [39]. This provides a rationale for combining retinoids with cytotoxic agents as discussed below. Some unwanted effects of differentiation have also been noticed. For example, RA-induced differentiation of human neuroblastoma cells increased the expression of the multi-drug resistance gene MDRI, suggesting that if retinoids are to be used in combination with cytotoxic agents then the agents should be selected based on their independence of MDR-mediated resistance [40,41].

Changes in Cell Phenotype Induced by Retinoids

Numerous reports have described a variety of phenotypic changes in tumour cells, and many of those changes could play a role in either growth inhibition or differentiation induction. Table 1 presents several structural and regulatory modulations that have been observed in various tumour cells induced to differentiate by retinoids or in response to retinoid treatment. It is well established that cell-cell communication is disrupted at early stages of carcinogenesis. Therefore, the ability of retinoids to enhance gap-junctional communication via increased expression of connexin 43 may be relevant for the chemopreventive activity of retinoids [42]. The interactions of cells with the extracellular matrix via cell surface components may be important for expression of tissue-specific genes and for preventing conversion of intraepithelial neoplasia to invasive malignant carcinoma. Retinoids induce the expression of various integrins in embryonal carcinoma [43] and in neuroblastoma cells [44], as well as the expression of matrix components such as laminin, proteoglycans, hyaluronic acid, collagen type IV in embryonal carcinoma cells [45]; some matrix proteins can also be induced in other cell types. Cell adhesion molecules (CAMs) that mediate cell-to-cell adhesion are also increased by retinoids [46]. Differentiation is often associated with changes in cell membrane structure resulting from alterations in lipid composition and glycolipid structure [47]. Such changes may influence membrane physicochemical properties and possibly the function of some membrane receptors for growth factors.

Mechanisms Underlying the Effects of Retinoids on the Growth and Differentiation of Tumour Cells

Although the ability of retinoids to inhibit proliferation and clonogenicity of malignant cells and modulate their differentiation *in vitro* is well documented as described above, the mechanism(s) responsible for these effects is not fully understood. The ability of retinoids to modulate gene expression is the most plausible mechanism by which they can modulate the differentiation and growth of malignant cells or suppress the progression of premalignant cells to neoplastic lesions by redirecting their differentiation. The identity of the genes that control the expression of the premalignant or the malignant phenotype is not known, however, the restoration of normal differentiation by retinoids may represent a part of a retinoid-dependent programme of gene expression that includes activation of intrinsic suppressor genes or inhibition of genes (e.g., oncogenes) that are required for maintenance of the malignant phenotype. Some of the effects of retinoids and the genes that may mediate these effects are presented in Table 1. Only limited evidence for direct regulation of the expression of these genes by retinoids is available. Important processes of signal transduction are modulated by retinoids. Thus, retinoids can either increase or decrease the expression of a large number of cell surface receptors for a variety of cytokines and growth factors. Their effects are often cell type specific and may reflect the cellular state of differentiation. A characteristic effect of retinoids is to subvert growth stimulatory signals mediated via different receptors. For example, RA has been reported to suppress the transcription of EGF-R in cervical carcinoma cells [48] and to decrease the protein tyrosine kinase activity of the receptor without decreasing its protein level in glioma cells [49]. The level of the related HER2/neu decreased on the surface of human breast carcinoma cells induced to differentiate with RA [50]. Another set of targets for retinoid modulation are the cytokines and growth factors. RA was found to decrease the level of TGF-α in human EC cells [51] and in breast carcinoma cells [52], thereby decreasing their growth. Other suppressive effects of retinoids on growth factor expression include the decreased level of IGF-I mRNA in glioma cells [53] and increased secretion by human breast carcinoma cells MCF-7 of IGF-binding proteins, which bind IGFs and prevent them from stimulating cell growth via IGF receptors [54]. Induction of the TGF-ß1 receptor expression and TGF-ß1 protein production in HL-60 cells by RA has been shown to generate an inhibitory autocrine loop [55]. In some neuroblastoma cells (e.g., SH-SY5Y), differentiation induction by retinoids may be mediated by increased expression of TrkB, a receptor for several neurotrophins. The addition of the neurotrophin BDNF to RA-treated cells induced TrkB phosphorylation and neuronal differentiation [56]. Retinoids were also reported to modulate the expression of various protooncogenes [57,58], suppressor genes [e.g. 59], and cell cycle-regulatory kinases [60] that are either reflecting the induction of a more differentiated phenotype or the reduced growth rate of the cells. Some of the changes occur within a few hours of treatment initiation and may therefore be related causally to subsequent events such as growth suppression or differentiation induction as was shown for the suppression of N-*myc* in neuroblastoma cells [61,62].

In addition to the effect of retinoids on cell surface-mediated signal reception, they also intervene with intracellular signalling via second messengers. Both increases and decreases have been reported in the level of protein kinases A and C. Neuronal differentiation of human EC cells was accompanied by increases in both pKA and pKC [63], and an increase in pKC-alpha was implicated in the induction of melanoma cell differentiation [64]. In contrast, neuronal differentiation of neuroblastoma cells was accompanied by a decreased level of pKC-alpha [65]. These results suggest that many of the effects of RA are cell type specific and cannot be generalised. It is still not clear how retinoids alter the expression of the above genes. Some of them may be regulated directly whereas others may be altered indirectly as a results of the initiation of a new gene expression programme or in response to an altered growth state.

To modulate gene expression retinoids must transmit signals to the cell nucleus. The mechanism of this signal transduction may involve both cytoplasmic and nuclear retinoid-binding proteins. These appear to play important roles in the series of events that are initiated with the uptake of a retinoid by a target cell and culminate in the modulation of gene transcription in the cell's nucleus.

As noted in the chapter by Zelent, several members of the large family of steroid and thyroid hormone receptors have been found to act as nuclear RA-binding proteins [2,3,10]. These receptors are retinoid-activated, DNA-binding, transacting transcription factors. Three RARs designated RAR-α, RAR-ß, and RAR-γ exhibit specific patterns of expression in the developing embryo as well as distinct distributions in adult tissues. Related nuclear RA receptors designated RXR-α, RXR-ß, and RXR-γ have been found to play an important role in the action of retinoids and other hormone receptors and transcription factors. Whereas the RARs bind all-*trans* RA and 9-*cis* RA, a natural RA metabolite, the RXRs bind only the latter retinoid. RXRs form heterodimers with RARs before binding to specific DNA sequences (RA response elements [RARE]) in the promoter regions of numerous retinoid-regulated genes [2-4,10]. RXRs can also heterodimerise with thyroid hormone receptors, the vitamin D3 receptor, the peroxisome proliferator-activated receptor, and the transcription factor COUP. The RA nuclear receptors may also interact antagonistically with components of other signal transaction pathways such as the AP-1 (*jun-fos*) transcription factor complex in stromelysin, collagenase and osteocalcin promoters, possibly by direct protein-protein interactions. Thus the regulation of a given gene by retinoids may depend on the relative concentrations of particular RARs, RXRs, the nature of the retinoic acid response elements (RAREs) in that gene, as well as on the presence of a number of other transcription factors.

Direct proof for the role of nuclear RA receptors in regulation of the growth inhibitory effect of retinoids or their effects on the differentiation programmes is available for only a few cases. The most compelling evidence in this regard is the demonstration by Collins et al. [66] that retroviral-mediated transduction of a wild-type RAR-α restored the response of an RA-resistant HL-60, possessing a mutant RAR-α, to the growth-inhibitory and differentiation-inducing effects of RA. The same group also demonstrated that a similar expression of transduced RAR-α in RA-resistant K562 cells, derived from a chronic myelogenous leukaemia patient at the blast crisis stage, which normally express a very low level of non-defective RAR-α, rendered the cells responsive to growth-inhibitory effects of RA. Treatment of squamous carcinoma cells with antisense oligonucleotides for the suppression of the expression of RAR-α resulted in inhibition of alkaline phosphatase induction by retinoids [67]. Other evidence includes the finding that the biological activity of several retinoids correlates well with their affinity for the nuclear receptors. That RARs play a role in embryonal carcinoma differentiation was concluded from studies that showed that a RA-non-responsive P19 subclone expressed an abundant truncated transcript [68] and that overexpression of an RAR-α, truncated in the ligand-binding domain, in F9 cells inhibited the RA inducibility of some genes (e.g., laminin B1, tissue plasminogen activator) without affecting the expression of Hox-1.3 and type IV collagen [69]. Both studies suggested that truncated receptors interfered with endogenous RARs in a negative dominant fashion to inhibit certain aspects of RA-induced differentiation.

Although the above results strongly support a direct role for RARs in mediating RA actions, the presence of an RAR is not sufficient to render a cell responsive to the growth-inhibitory or differentiation-inducing effects of retinoids. For example, RAR-α is expressed by most human leukaemias (fresh cells and cell lines) regardless of their responsiveness to RA [70]. We found that an RA-resistant mutant of melanoma cells does not differ from sensitive wild-type clone in constitutive expression of RAR-α and RAR-γ, in the induction of RAR-ß [71], and in the activation of transcription from RAR-ß RARE. Similar results were found for RAR's constitutive expression and inducibility in murine PCC4aza1R embryonal carcinoma cells and 2 RA-resistant mutants derived from them. It appears therefore that RARs may be necessary but not sufficient for mediating the effects of retinoids on cell growth and differentiation.

Resistance to Effects of Retinoids

Malignant cells that are resistant to the growth-inhibitory effects of retinoids *in vitro* have been described. Such cells have been found to occur among tumour cell lines screened for responses to retinoids [1] or isolated by several methods: a) mutagenesis followed by selection for colony formation in agarose [72], b) continuous growth in the presence of retinol [73], or retinoic acid [66], c) transfection of a truncated nuclear RA receptor that acted as a negative dominant inhibitor of response [69], d) immortalisation by human papilloma virus (HPV) [74], and e) found to occur spontaneously [68]. The mechanisms of resistance to retinoids are not fully understood, however, several possibilities have emerged from recent studies. The aberrant expression, structure, or function of nuclear RA receptors appears to be one of the mechanisms of RA resistance [66,68]. RA-resistant HL-60 cells were found to contain a mutant RAR-α with low affinity for binding RA [66]. Similarly, RA-resistant embryonal carcinoma cell lines were found to either express a truncated form of RAR-α [68] or to have lost expression of RXR-α [75].

Other mechanisms for retinoid resistance have been described. Thus, the immortalisation of human keratinocytes by human papillomavirus 16 E6/E7 has led to resistance to the suppressive effect of retinoids on squamous cell differentiation compared with normal keratinocytes [74]. Interestingly, HPV-immortalised keratinocytes exhibited increased sensitivity to the growth-inhibitory effect of retinoids [76], indicating that in such cells RA effects on cell growth and on differentiation may be independent.

Retinoid resistance may develop in responsive cells via changes in signal transduction, autocrine responses and oncogene expression. In some neuroblastoma cells RA resistance is related to RA-induced expression of insulin-like growth factor (IGF) II, which is a major growth factor for these cells; the increased expression of this factor apparently counteracts the growth suppression, neurite outgrowth and apoptosis effects of RA [77]. In human ovarian teratocarcinoma PA-1 cells, RA-resistance of selected clones was associated with the presence of an activated N-*ras* and tumorigenicity [78]. Interestingly, selection of melanoma cells for resistance to 8-bromo-cyclic AMP-induced growth inhibition resulted in the isolation of clones that were cross-resistant to RA [79]. Resistance to RA could be reversed by agents that elevate intracellular cyclic AMP levels in neuroblastoma [80]. This effect may be related to the suggestion that cAMP regulates some steps in the RA signal transduction pathway [79]. The resistance of HL-60 cells to the differentiating effect of RA could be reversed by interferon-γ [81].

Inhibitory Effects of Retinoids on Tumorigenicity and Metastatic Propensity of Cultured Tumour Cells

The relevance of the growth-inhibitory and differentiation-inducing effects of retinoids in cultured cells *in vitro* to the clinical application of retinoids is of major importance. Studies with experimental animal models have afforded some insight into the effects of retinoids on tumour growth and metastasis. Most of the effects of retinoids on the growth and differentiation of tumour cells are reversible upon cessation of treatment; therefore, pretreatment of tumour cells *in vitro* before injecting them into syngeneic or immunocompromised mice has usually failed to inhibit tumour formation. However, in the case of human teratocarcinoma NT2, pretreatment *in vitro* resulted in irreversible differentiation and loss of tumorigenicity [51]. Murine F9 embryonal carcinoma cells did not lose tumorigenicity after *in vitro* pretreatment, however, their growth *in vivo* was suppressed and their differentiation was enhanced by intratumoural injection of RA [37] or by feeding the tumour-bearing mice with retinoids [38].

Several reports indicate that retinoids modulate tumour cell invasion and metastasis at various stages [for review and references see 82]. Pretreatment of tumour cells including human breast carcinoma, murine melanomas, and squamous cell carcinoma, with RA or 13-*cis* RA *in vitro* suppressed their metastatic potential analysed as organ colonisation following intravenous tumour cell injection. Unlike the above cell types, pretreatment of F9 cells with RA resulted in a moderate suppression of liver colonisation; however, the RA-treated cells formed lung tumours whereas the untreated cells formed liver colonies. Thus, RA treatment altered the organ colonisation specificity of F9 cells from liver to lung. Due to the reversible nature of retinoid effects the result of pretreatment with retinoids on experimental metastasis probably reflects alterations in early events in lung colonisation such as adhesion to endothelial cells or extracellular matrix at the site of implantation. To maintain the effect of retinoids they have to be administered to the host after injection of the tumour cells. Indeed, when human MDA-MB-231 breast carcinoma cells were treated *in vitro* with retinol and then injected i.v. into nude mice, which were subsequently treated with retinol intragastrically daily for 4 weeks, the treated mice developed considerably fewer lung metastases than did the control mice. These results demonstrated that the continuous exposure of the tumour cells to retinol suppressed their *in-vivo* lung colonisation potential. The ability of retinoids to suppress spontaneous metastasis resulting from the spread of tumour cells from a subcutaneous primary site has been demonstrated in several experimental systems and found to result in part from stimulation of host immune response via T cell-dependent responses as well as from a direct effect on tumour cells. The synthetic retinoid trimethymethoxyphenyl analogue of ethyl retinoate (TMMPER) administered intragastrically decreased the incidence of metastasis of immunogenic murine tumour cells in syngeneic mice but had no effect on non-immunogenic tumours of the same type. The direct effects of retinoids on tumour metastasis were demonstrated in congenitally athymic nude mice, which were inoculated s.c. with hamster melanoma cells and then fed with 13-*cis* RA, 2-hydroxyethyl retinamide (2-HER), or 4-hydroxyphenyl retinamide (4-HPR) at different doses. This treatment reduced the incidence of metastases.

Several mechanisms may account for the antimetastatic activity of retinoids. These include modulation of cell surface glycoconjugates [83], cell adhesion, production of matrix degrading enzymes [84,85], migration [86], and invasion [85]. Many of these may directly or indirectly have an impact on the metastatic potential of the tumour cells. In addition, retinoids may affect the host by inhibiting angiogenesis [87,88] and consequently reduce metastasis. RA inhibited the migration of mouse melanoma cells by suppressing the production of a cell surface receptor for motility factor in human and in mouse melanoma cells and prevented the enhancement of motility [85,86]. Retinoids inhibited the invasion of lung carcinoma, mammary carcinoma and melanoma through basement membrane. However, a few tumour cell lines responded in an opposite manner and their invasiveness increased after RA treatment. Retinoids modulate the levels of interstitial collagenases and type IV collagenase [84,85], and stromelysin [89]. In the case of collagenase the levels of enzyme protein and mRNA were decreased and it was suggested that retinoids interfere with the transcription of the collagenase gene by inhibiting the ability of c-*jun* to bind to the AP-1 site found in the collagenase promoter [90]. The decreased level of collagenase in RA-treated cells resulted in diminished ability of cultured human lung A549 carcinoma cells, rat mammary 13762NF carcinoma cells and human A375 melanoma cells to degrade purified type IV collagen, human amnion BM, or BM produced by cultured endothelial cells.

Effects of Retinoids in Combination with Other Agents

Extensive studies were carried out with the myeloid leukaemia cell line HL-60 in order to define the efficacy of combinations of retinoids and other agents [91]. Such studies have demonstrated additive or synergistic effects of retinoids and the following agents: dimethylsulphoxide, dimethylformamide, hexamethyl–enebisacetamide, butyrate, tiazofurin, tumour necrosis factor-α, 6-thiguanine, 5-aza-2'-deoxycytidine, actinomycin, granulocyte colony-stimulating factor and IL-6. Studies with embryonal carcinoma have shown that a combination of RA and cyclic AMP or cAMP elevating agents induce a pathway of endodermal differentiation distinct from that induced by RA alone. The combination of RA and tamoxifen was found to be more effective in suppressing the growth of human breast carcinoma cells than either agent alone [92]. In neuroblastoma cells, RA augmented the differentiation-inducing effect of cAMP and interferon-alpha and showed enhanced activity with cisplatin. Because the combination of 13-*cis* RA has been used successfully in several clinical trials, the nature of their interaction is of particular interest.

The efficacy of the combination of IFNs (mostly IFN-α and IFN-γ) and retinoids (mostly RA) in induction of differentiation and growth inhibition was detected initially *in vitro* in established leukaemia cell lines (e.g., HL60, U937). The effects of IFNs and retinoids were either additive or synergistic, depending on the cell system evaluated; moreover, distinct differentiation pathways could be stimulated in different cell types. Furthermore, IFN-α restored responsiveness to RA in RA-resistant HL60 cells [81]. Likewise, IFN-γ restored responsiveness to RA in RA-resistant v-*myc* expressing U937 cells. Further studies with fresh leukaemic cells from AML patients treated in short-term cultures with IFNs and RA also demonstrated synergistic growth inhibition and differentiation induction with the combination. In addition, increased inhibition of clonal growth and differentiation was observed after *in vitro* RA treatment of cells from patients treated with IFN-α *in vivo*. Additive or synergistic growth inhibition of various human tumour cell lines *in vitro* was reported for the combination of IFN-α or IFN-γ and RA or other retinoids. These effects were sometimes also associated with differentiation induction, particularly in neuroblastoma cells. Tumour cell types in which the combination of the two agents showed greater growth inhibition than each agent alone included breast carcinoma, osteosarcoma, ovarian carcinoma, SCC, neuroblastoma, non-small cell lung carcinoma, and cervical carcinoma [93]. Furthermore, the growth of human neuroblastoma tumours in nude mice was inhibited synergistically by the combination of IFN-γ and RA. These combined effects of IFNs and retinoids may result from activation of the same genes or distinct genes, depending on the cell type. For example, both agents induce 2-5-OASE gene transcription in some cells. In other cells, one agent can potentiate the effect of the other by different mechanisms. For example, RA increased the binding of ^{125}I-labeled IFN-α to various tumour cell lines by increasing the number of receptors. RA also stabilised 2-5-OASE mRNA induced by IFN-α [94]. By contrast, IFN-γ did not alter the level of cellular RA-binding proteins and IFN-α did not affect the levels of nuclear RARs in several tumour cell lines. The agents may work through different mechanisms as well. For example, human neuroblastoma cells are induced to differentiate by either agent alone, but the combination of agents leads to synergistic effects, probably via distinct mechanisms as indicated by the finding that RA increases inositol 1,4,5-trisphosphate and 1,2-diacylglycerol (PKC activator), whereas IFN-γ has no effect on the level of these second messengers.

Conclusions

Cancer development and progression are closely associated with disturbed regulation of cell growth and differentiation. One of the non-cytotoxic developmental therapeutic approaches to overcome these abnormalities is the identification of agents that can restore normal regulatory mechanisms to premalignant or malignant cells, thereby reversing premalignant lesions and suppressing the growth of tumours. Although retinoids exhibit the required effects *in vitro*, there are only limited successes to date in cancer prevention or treatment. Clearly, there is a great deal of enthusiasm among researchers in the field of retinoids, as rapid developments concerning new genes regulated by retinoids and novel aspects of their mechanism of action on gene expression continue to be reported at an incredible rate. However, there still exists a large gap between the findings in model systems and cultured cells and the translation of these findings to the clinical application of retinoids in cancer prevention and therapy of solid tumours. Closure of this gap requires collaboration between basic and clinical researchers.

Acknowledgement

Research in the author's laboratory was supported in part by USPHS grant PO1-CA52051 from the NCI.

REFERENCES

1 Lotan R: Effects of vitamin A and its analogs (retinoids) on normal and neoplastic cells. Biochim Biophys Acta Rev Cancer 1980 (605):33-91

2 DeLuca LM: Retinoids and their receptors in differentiation, embryogenesis and neoplasia. FASEB J 1991 (5):2924-1933

3 Lotan R and Clifford JL: Nuclear receptors for retinoids: mediators of retinoid effects on normal and malignant cells. Biomed Pharmacother 1991 (45):145-156

4 Gudas LJ: Retinoids, retinoid-responsive genes, cell differentiation, and cancer. Cell Growth Diff 1992 (3):655-662

5 Jetten AM, Nervi C, Vollberg TM: Control of squamous differentiation in tracheobronchial and epidermal epithelial cells: role of retinoids. JNCI Monograph 1992 (13):93-100

6 Smith MA, Parkinson DR, Cheson BD, Friedman MA: Retinoids in cancer therapy. J Clin Oncol 1992 (10): 839-864

7 Packer L (ed) Methods in Enzymology: Retinoids. Academic Press, Orlando 1991

8 Morriss-Kay G (ed) Retinoids in Normal Development and Teratogenesis. Oxford University Press, New York 1992

9 Hong WK and Lotan R: Retinoids in Oncology. Marcel Dekker, Inc, New York 1993

10 Sporn MB, Roberts AB, Goodman DS: The Retinoids. Biology. Chemistry. and Medicine. Raven Press, New York1994

11 Amos B and Lotan R: Retinoid sensitive cells and cell lines. In: Packer L (ed) Methods in Enzymology: Retinoids. Academic Press, Orlando 1991 pp 217-225

12 Lotan R, Lotan D, Sacks P: Inhibition of tumor cell growth by retinoids. In: Packer L (ed) Methods in Enzymology: Retinoids. Academic Press, Orlando 1990 pp 100-110

13 Schroder EW, Rapaport E, Kabcenell AK, Black PH: Growth Inhibitory and stimulatory effects of retinoic acid on murine 3T3 cells. Proc Natl Acad Sci USA 1982 (79):1549-1552

14 Butler WB and Fontana JA: Responses to retinoic acid of tamoxifen-sensitive and resistant sublines of human breast cancer cell line MCF-7. Cancer Res 1992 (52):6164-6167

15 Lotan R, Lotan D, Kadoury A: Comparison of retinoic acid effects on anchorage-dependent growth, anchorage-independent growth and fibrinolytic activity of neoplastic cells. Exp Cell Res 1982 (141):79-86

16 Meyskens FL Jr and Salmon SE: Inhibition of human melanoma colony formation by retinoids. Cancer Res 1979 (39):4055-4057

17 Meyskens FL Jr, Alberts DS, Salmon SE: Effect of 13-cis-retinoic acid and 4-hydroxyphenyl-all-trans-retinamide on human tumor colony formation in soft agar. Int J Cancer 1983 (32):295-299

18 Cowan JD, Von Hoff DD, Dinesman A, Clark G: Use of a human tumor cloning system to screen retinoids for antineoplastic activity. Cancer 1983 (51):92-96

19 Piacentini M, Annicchiarico-Petruzzelli M, Oliverio S, Piredda L, Biedler JI, Melino E: Phenotype-specific "tissue" transglutaminase regulation in human neuroblastoma cells in response to retinoic acid: correlation with cell death by apoptosis. Int J Cancer 1992 (52):271-278

20 Davies PJA, Stein JP, Chiocca EA, Basilon IP, Gentile V, Thomazy V, Fesus L: Retinoid-regulated expression of transglutaminases: links to the biochemistry of programmed cell death. In: Morriss-Kay G (ed) Relinoids in Normal Development and Teratogenesis. Oxford University Press, Oxford 1992 pp 249-263

21 Jiang H and Kochhar DM: Induction of tissue transglutaminase and apoptosis by retinoic acid in the limb bud. Teratology 1992 (46):333-340

22 Martin SJ, Bradley JG, Cotter TG: HL-60 cells induced to differentiate towards neutrophils subsequently die via apoptosis. Clin Exp Immunol 1990 (79):448-453

23 Chomienne C, Barbey S, Balitrand N, Degos L, Sachs L: Regulation of Bcl-2 and cell death by all-trans retinoic acid in acute promyelocytic leukemic cells. Proc Amer Assoc Cancer Res 1992 (33):41, abst 246

24 Delia D, Aiello A, Lombardi L, Pellici PG, Grignani F, Grignani F, Formelli F, Menard S, Costa A, Veronesi U, Pierotti MA: N-(4-hydroxyphenyl)retinamide induces apoptosis of malignant hemopoietic cell lines including those unresponsive to retinoic acid. Cancer Res 1993 (53):6036-6041

25 Roberts AB and Sporn MB: Mechanistic inter-relationships between two superfamilies: the steroid/retinoid receptors and transforming growth factor-ß. Cancer Surv 1992 (14):204-220

26 Lotan R: Retinoids and squamous cell differentiation. In: Hong WK and Lotan R (eds) Retinoids in Oncology. Marcel Dekker, New York 1993 pp 43-72

27 Strickland S, Smith KK, Marotti KR: Hormonal induction of differentiation in teratocarcinoma stem cells: generation of parietal endoderm by retinoic acid and dibutyryl cAMP. Cell 1980 (21):347-355

28 Andrews PW: Retinoic acid induces neuronal differentiation of a cloned human embryonal carcinoma cell line in vitro. Dev Biol 1984 (103):285-293

29 McBurney MW, Jones-Villeneuve EM, Edwards MK, Anderson PJ: Control of muscle and neuronal differentiation in a cultured embryonal carcinoma cell line. Nature 1982 (299):165-167

30 Breitman TR, Selonick SE, Collins SJ: Induction of differentiation of the human promyelocytic leukemia cell line (HL60) by retinoic acid. Proc Natl Acad Sci USA 1980 (77):2936-2940

31 Damjanov I, Horvat B, Gibas Z: Retinoic acid-induced differentiation of the developmentally pluripotent human germ cell tumor-derived cell line, NCCIT. Lab Invest 1993 (68):220-232

32 Boncinelli E, Simeone A, Acampora D, Mavilio F: HOX gene activation by retinoic acid. Trends Genet 1991 (7):329-334

33 Luscher B, Mitchell PJ, Williams T, Tjian R: Regulation of transcription factor AP-2 by the morphogen retinoic acid and by second messengers. Genes Dev 1989 (3):1507- 1517

34 Lucke-Huhle C and Herrlich P: Retinoic acid-induced differentiation prevents gene amplification in teratocarcinoma stem cells. Int J Cancer 1991 (47): 461-465
35 Imaizumi M and Breitman TR: Retinoic acid-induced differentiation of the human promyelocytic leukemia cell line, HL-60, and fresh human leukemia cells in primary culture: a model for differentiation inducing therapy of leukemia. Eur J Haematol 1987 (38):289-302
36 Muench MO, Guy Z, Moore MA: Ex vivo differentiation therapy as a method of leukemic cell purging in murine bone marrow expansion cultures. Cancer Res 1992 (52):6576-6582
37 Speers WC and Altmann M: Chemically induced differentiation of murine embryonal carcinomas in vivo transplantation of differentiated tumors. Cancer Res 1984 (44):2129-2135
38 McCue PA, Thomas RS, Schroeder D, Gubler M, Sherman MI: Effects of dietary retinoids upon growth and differentiation of tumors derived from several murine embryonal carcinoma cell lines. Cancer Res 1988 (48):3772-3779
39 Guchelaar HJ, Timmer-Bosscha H, Dam-Meiring A, Uges DR, Oosterhuis JW, de Vries E. G, Mulder NH: Enhancement of cisplatin and etoposide cytotoxicity after all-trans retinoic-acid-induced cellular differentiation of a murine embryonal carcinoma cell line. Int J Cancer 1993 (55):442-447
40 Bates SE, Mickley LA, Chen YN, Richert N, Rudick J, Biedler JL, Fojo AT: Expression of drug resistance gene in human neuroblastoma cell lines: modulation by retinoic acid-induced differentiation. Mol Cell Biol 1989 (9):4337-4344
41 Ferrandis E and Benard J: Activation of the human MDR1 gene promoter in differentiated neuroblasts. Int J Cancer 1993 (54):987-991
42 Rogers M, Berestecky JM, Hossain MZ, Guo HM, Kadle R, Nicholson BJ, Bertram JS: Retinoid-enhanced gap junctional communication is achieved by increased levels of connexin 43 mRNA and protein. Mol Carcinogenesis 1990 (3):335-343
43 Dedhar S, Robertson K, Gray V: Induction of expression of the alpha v beta I and alpha v beta 3 integrin heterodimers during retinoic acid-induced neuronal differentiation of murine embryonal carcinoma cells. J Biol Chem 1991 (266):21846-21852
44 Rossino P, Defilippi P, Silengo L, Tarone G: Upregulation of the integrin alpha I/beta I in human neuroblastoma cells differentiated by retinoic acid: correlation with increased neurite outgrowth response to laminin. Cell Regul 1991 (2):1021-1033
45 Gudas LJ, Grippo JF, Kim KW, LaRosa GJ, Stoner CM: The regulation of the expression of genes encoding basement membrane proteins during the retinoic acid-associated differentiation of murine teratocarcinoma cells. Ann NY Acad Sci 1990 (580):245-251
46 Bouillon M, Tessier P, Boulianne R, Destrempe R, Audette M: Regulation by retinoic acid of ICAM-I expression on human tumor cell lines. Biochim Biophys Acta 1991 (1097):95-102
47 Andrews PW, Nudelman E, Hakomori S, Fenderson BA: Different patterns of glycolipid antigens are expressed following differentiation of TERA-2 human embryonal carcinoma cells induced by retinoic acid, hexamethylene bisacetamide (HMBA) or bromodeoxyuridine (BUdR). Differentiation 1990 (43):131-138
48 Zheng ZS, Polakowska R, Johnson A, Goldsmith LA: Transcriptional control of epidermal growth factor receptor by retinoic acid. Cell Growth Diff 1992 (3):225-232
49 Steck PA, Hadi A, Lotan R, Yung WK: Inhibition of epidermal growth factor receptor activity by retinoic acid in glioma cells. J Cell Biochem 1990 (42):83-94
50 Bacus SS, Kiguchi, K, Chin, D, King CR, Huberman E: Differentiation of cultured human breast cancer cells (AU-565 and MCF-7) associated with loss of cell surface HER-2/neu antigen. Mol Carcinogenesis 1990 (3):350-362
51 Dmitrovsky E, Moy D, Miller WH, Jr, Li A, Masui H: Retinoic acid causes a decline in TGF-alpha expression, cloning effciency, and tumorigenicity in a human embryonal cancer cell line. Oncogene Res 1990 (5):233-239
52 Fontana JA, Nervi C, Shao ZM, Jetten AM: Retinoid antagonism of estrogen-responsive transforming growth factor alpha and pS2 gene expression in breast carcinoma cells. Cancer Res 1992 (52):3938-3945
53 Lowe WL, Meyer T, Karpen CW, Lorentzen LR: Regulation of insulin-like growth factor I production in rat C6 glioma cells: possible role as an autocrine/paracrine growth factor. Endocrinology 1992 (130):2683-2689
54 Fontana JA, Burrows-Mezu A, Clemmons DR, LeRoith D: Retinoid modulation of insulin-like growth factor-binding proteins and inhibition of breast carcinoma proliferation. Endocrinology 1991 (128): 1115-1122
55 Falk LA, De Benedetti F, Lohrey N, Birchenall-Roberts MC, Ellingsworth LW, Faltynek CR, Ruscetti FW: Induction of transforming growth factor-beta 1 (TGF-beta 1), receptor expression and TGF-beta-1 protein production in retinoic acid treated HL-60 cells: possible TGF-beta-1-mediated autocrine inhibition. Blood 1991 (77):1248-1255
56 Kaplan DR, Matsumoto K, Lucarelli E, Thiele C: Induction of TrkB by retinoic acid mediates biologic responsiveness to BDNF and differentiation of human neuroblastoma cells. Neuron 1993 (11):321-331
57 Dean M, Levine RA, Campisi J: C-myc regulation during retinoic acid-induced differentiation of F9 cells is posttranscriptional and associated with growth arrest. Mol Cell Biol 1986 (6):518-524
58 Busam KJ, Roberts AB, Sporn MB: Inhibition of mitogen-induced c-fos expression in melanoma cells by retinoic acid involves the serum response element. J Biol Chem 1992 (267):19971-19977
59 Slack RS, Hamel PA, Bladon TS, Gill RM, McBurney MW: Regulated expression of the retinoblastoma gene in differentiating embryonal carcinoma cells. Oncogene 1993 (8):1585-1591
60 Gaetano C, Matsumoto K, Thiele CJ: Retinoic acid negatively regulates p34cdc2 expression during human neuroblastoma differentiation. Cell Growth Differ 1991 (2):487-493

61 Thiele CJ, Reynolds PC, Israel MA: Decreased expression of N-*myc* precedes retinoic acid-induced morphological differentiation of human neuroblastoma. Nature 1985 (313):404-406

62 Thiele CJ, Deutsch LA, Israel MA: The expression of multiple proto-oncogenes is differentially regulated during retinoic acid induced maturation of human neuroblastoma cell lines. Oncogene 1988 (3):281-288

63 Abraham I, Sampson KE, Powers EA, Mayo JK, Ruff VA, Leach KL (1991): Increased PKA and PKC activities accompany neuronal differentiation of NT2/DI cells. J Neurosci Res 1991 (28):29-39

64 Gruber JR, Ohno S, Niles RM: Increased expression of protein kinase C alpha plays a key role in retinoic acid-induced melanoma differentiation. J Biol Chem 1992 (267):13356-13360

65 Tonini GP, Parodi MT, Di Martino D, Varesio L: Expression of protein kinase C-alpha (PKC-alpha) and MYCN mRNAs in human neuroblastoma cells and modulation during morphological differentiation induced by retinoic acid. FEBS Leu 1991 (280):221-224

66 Collins SJ, Robertson KA, Mueller L: Retinoic acid-induced granulocytic differentiation of HL-60 myeloid leukemia cells is mediated directly through the retinoic acid receptor (RAR-α). Mol Cell Biol 1990 (10):2154-2163

67 Cope FO and Wille JJ (1989): Retinoid receptor antisense DNAs inhibit alkaline phosphatase induction and clonogenicity in malignant keratinocytes. Proc Natl Acad Sci USA 1989 (86):5590-5594

68 Pratt MAC, Kralova J, McBurney MW: A dominant negative mutation of the alpha retinoic acid receptor gene in a retinoic acid-non-responsive embryonal carcinoma cell. Mol Cell Biol 1990 (10):6445-6453

69 Espeseth AS, Murphy SP, Linney E: Retinoic acid receptor expression vector inhibits differentiation of F9 embryonal carcinoma cells. Genes Dev 1989 (3):1647-1656

70 Gallagher RE, Said F, Pua I, Papenhausen PR, Paietta E, Wiernik PH: Expression of retinoic acid receptor-α mRNA in human leukemia cells with variable responsiveness to retinoic acid. Leukemia 1989 (3):789-795

71 Clifford JL, Petkovich M, Chambon P, Lotan R: Induction by ß-all-trans retinoic acid (RA) of nuclear retinoic acid receptor ß (RAR-ß) in murine melanoma cells. Mol Endocrinol 1989 (4):1546-1555

72 Lotan R, Stolarsky T, Lotan D: Isolation and analysis of melanoma cell mutants resistant to the anti-proliferative action of retinoic acid. Cancer Res 1983 (43):2868-2875

73 Halter SA, Fraker LD, Parl F, Bradley R, Briggs R: Selective isolation of human breast carcinoma cells resistant to the growth-inhibitory effects of retinol. Nutr Cancer 1990 (14):43-56

74 Merrick DT, Gown AM, Halbert CL, Blanton RA, McDougall JK: Human papillomavirus-immortalized keratinocytes are resistant to the effects of retinoic acid on terminal differentiation. Cell Growth Diff 1993 (4):831-840

75 Kurie JM, Buck J, Eppinger TM, Moy D, Dmitrovsky E: 9-cis and all-trans retinoic acid induce a similar phenotype in human teratocarcinoma cells. Differentiation 1993 (54):123-129

76 Pirisi L, Batova A, Jenkins GR, Hodam JR, Creek KE: Increased sensitivity of human keratinocytes immortalized by human papillomavirus type 16 DNA to growth control by retinoids. Cancer Res 1992 (52):187-193

77 Melino G, Stephanou A, Annicchiarico-Petruzzelli M, Knight RA, Finazzi-Agro A, Lightman SL: Modulation of IGF-2 expression during growth and differentiation of human neuroblastoma cells: retinoic acid may induce IGF-2. Neurosci Lett 1993 (151):187-191

78 Tainsky MA, Yim SO, Krizman DB, Kannan P, Chiao PJ, Mukhopadhyay T, Buettner R: Modulation of differentiation in PA-1 human teratocarcinoma cells after N-*ras* oncogene-induced tumorigenicity. Oncogene 1991 (6):1575-1582

79 Niles RM and Loewy B: B16 mouse melanoma cells selected for resistance to cyclic AMP-mediated growth inhibition are cross-resistant to retinoic acid-induced growth inhibition. J Cell Physiol 1991 (147): 176-181

80 Abemayor E: The effects of retinoic acid on the in vitro and in vivo growth of neuroblastoma cells. Laryngoscope 1992 (102):1133-1149

81 Grant. S, Bhalla K, Weinstein IB, Pestka S, Mileno MD, Fisher PB: Recombinant human interferon sensitizes resistant myeloid leukemic cells to induction of terminal differentiation. Biochem Biophys Res Commun 1985 (130):379-388

82 Lotan R: Inhibitory effects of retinoids on tumor cell invasion and metastasis. In: Rabes HM, Peters PE, Munk K (eds) Metastasis: Basic Research and Clinical Applications. Contributions to Oncology, Vol 44. Karger, Basel 1992 pp 154-175

83 Amos B, Deutsch V, Lotan R: Modulation by all-trans retinoic acid of glycoprotein glycosylation in murine melanoma cells: enhancement of fucosyl- and galactosyl-transferase activities. Cancer Biochem Biophys 1990 (11):31-43

84 Nakajima M, Lotan D, Baig MM, Carralero RM, Wood WR, Hendrix MJ, Lotan R: Inhibition by retinoic acid of type IV collagenolysis and invasion through reconstituted basement membrane by metastatic rat mammary adenocarcinoma cells. Cancer Res 1989 (49):1698-1706

85 Hendrix MCJ, Wood WR, Seftor EA, Lotan D, Nakajima M, Misiorowski RL, Seftor REB, Stetler-Stevenson WG, Bevacqua SJ, Liotta LA, Sobel ME, Raz A, Lotan R: Retinoic acid inhibition of human melanoma cell invasion through a reconstituted basement membrane and its relation to decreases in the expression of proteolytic enzymes and motility factor receptor. Cancer Res 1990 (50):4121-4130

86 Lotan R, Amos, B, Watanabe H, Raz A: Suppression of melanoma cell motility factor receptor expression by retinoic acid. Cancer Res 1992 (52):4878-4884

87 Ingber D and Folkman J: Inhibition of angiogenesis through modulation of collagen metabolism. Lab Invest 1988 (59):44-51

88 Oikawa T, Hirotani K, Nakamura O, Shudo K, Hiragun A, Iwaguchi T: A highly potent antiangiogenic activity of retinoids. Cancer Lett 1989 (48): 157-162

89 Nicholson RC, Mader S, Nagpal S, Leid M, Rochette-Egly C, Chambon P: Negative regulation of the rat stromelysin gene promoter by retinoic acid is mediated by an AP1 binding site. EMBO J 1990 (9): 4443-4454
90 Schule R, Rangarajan P, Yang N, Kliewer S, Ransone LJ, Boland J, Verma IM, Evans RM: Retinoic acid is a negative regulator of AP-1-responsive genes. Proc Natl Acad Sci USA 1991 (88):6092-6096
91 Breitman TR and He RY: Combinations of retinoic acid with either sodium butyrate, dimethyl sulfoxide, or hexamethylene bisacetamide synergistically induce differentiation of the human myeloid leukemia cell line HL60. Cancer Res 1990 (50):6268-6273
92 Fontana JA: Interaction of retinoids and tamoxifen on the inhibition of human mammary carcinoma cell proliferation. Exp Cell Biol 1987 (55):136-144
93 Bollag W, Peck R, Frey JR: Inhibition of proliferation by retinoids and cytokines and their combination in four human transformed epithelial cell lines. Cancer Lett 1992 (62):167- 172
94 Higuchi T, Hannigan GE, Malkin D, Yeger H, Williams BR: Enhancement by retinoic acid and dibutyryl cyclic adenosine 3':5'-monophosphate of the differentiation and gene expression of human neuroblastoma cells induced by interferon. Cancer Res 1991 (51):3958-3964

Retinoids and Embryos

Gillian Morriss-Kay

Department of Human Anatomy, University of Oxford, South Parks Road, Oxford OX1 3QX, United Kingdom

The highly controlled manner of growth and change in embryos appears at first sight to be a world apart from the apparent disorder of cancer. However, the enormous variety of biological processes within a single embryo may offer some useful parallels with the molecular and cellular basis of oncogenesis. The control of retinoid levels within embryos, and the effects of altered retinoid levels on development, are particularly relevant in this respect.

This chapter is organised into 3 sections. First I will make some basic introductory remarks about embryology; next I will give an overview of the distribution of retinoic acid receptors and retinoid binding proteins in embryos, with some functional interpretations; finally I will give some examples of the effects of altered retinoid levels on the developmental programme of specific cell populations. All of the work discussed and referred to is from studies on mammalian embryos (mainly mouse and rat). Many experimental studies on retinoids have used avian and amphibian embryos (see Zelent, this volume, for references). However, just as different cell lines and different tumours have specific responses to retinoids, so do embryos of different classes of vertebrates. Mammalian embryos are therefore the best model for studies aimed at shedding light on human development, and may also be most relevant when looking for developmental parallels with human cancers.

Embryology: Some Basic Principles

Embryogenesis involves 3 major processes: growth, differentiation and morphogenesis. The first two of these are of obvious importance in the context of oncology, and the third should not be dismissed as of "in house" interest to embryologists only. Morphogenesis includes processes such as the transformation of epithelial tissues into migratory cell populations; the migratory cells, which are undifferentiated, move to new positions, so that they are able to make new contacts and interactions with other embryonic tissues. Embryonic tissue interactions involve a dialogue between two adjacent cell populations, often an epithelium and a mesenchymal tissue, and the intervening extracellular matrix plays a crucial role [1]. The result of this dialogue is a new local programme of gene expression leading to highly controlled patterns of growth, morphogenesis and differentiation. Morphogenesis can occur in the absence of growth [2], but in general all three of these processes play coordinated roles in the generation of developmental change. Terminal differentiation normally means that cells leave the cell cycle permanently, but differentiation in embryos is a gradual process, and patterns of gene expression indicative of specific cell lineages occur in cell populations that are still undergoing mitosis.

Neurulation (formation of the neural tube, i.e., the future brain and spinal cord) is a good example of a developmental process illustrating the harmonization of growth, morphogenesis and differentiation. The pattern of growth within the neuroepithelium is strictly controlled as it changes shape to form the neural tube [3]; many of the genes whose regional patterns of expression establish the future regional structure within the brain are expressed while the cranial neural folds are still open [4]; in the spinal cord, the process of differentiation into neurones and non-neuronal cell types begins as soon as the neural tube closes [5].

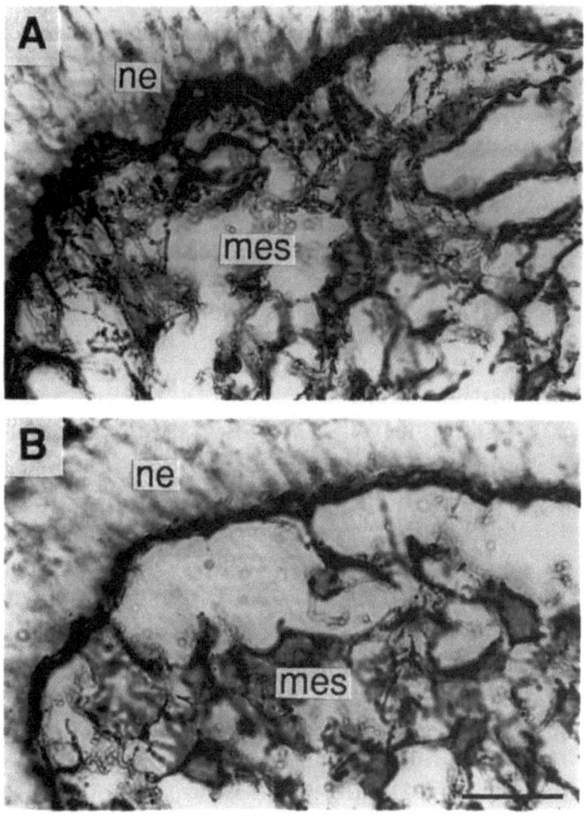

Fig. 1. Transverse section of cranial neural folds, day 9 rat embryo, cultured for 3 hours in (A) addition-free medium and (B) medium containing 0.25 μg/ml (8.3×10^{-7} M) retinoic acid. Immunohistochemical staining shows the presence of heparan sulphate proteoglycan (HSPG) in the mesenchyme (mes) and basement membrane of the neuroepithelium (ne), and in material between the basement membrane and mesenchymal cells. Within 3 hours of exposure of the embryos to retinoic acid much of the HSPG is lost, particularly from the material immediately beneath the basement membrane. Subsequently, patterns of gene expression, growth and morphogenesis within the neuroepithelium are abnormal (see [6] for details). Bar line = 20 μm

Neurulation is also typical of a morphogenetic process that involves an interaction between two adjacent tissues, together with their associated extracellular matrix. The two tissues are the neuroepithelium and its underlying mesenchyme; the mesenchyme is derived from cells which have migrated to this position from the caudally situated primitive streak, in which they were converted from an epithelial to a mesenchymal population. The basement membrane of the neuroepithelium, and the extracellular matrix of the underlying mesenchymal tissue, are both rich in heparan sulphate proteoglycan (HSPG) [6]: removal of this material by means of intra-amniotic injection of heparitinase inhibits neurulation [7]. Neurulation is delayed and sometimes inhibited by exposure of the embryos to retinoic acid, and this effect is correlated with the loss of much of the immunohistochemical staining for HSPG [6] (Fig.1).

Developmental processes are governed by complex sequences of gene expression. Many of the developmentally important genes encode transcription factors, or secreted proteins that influence transcription in responding cells, so it is easy to appreciate that the expression of one gene can lead to the transcription or repression of another, in the same or an adjacent cell. The molecular genetics of development are understood in some detail in the fruit-fly, *Drosophila,* where it is clear that developmental pattern is the result of coordinated cascades of gene expression. For instance, the segmented structure of the insect body results from a combination of genes whose products, and their interactions, control pattern and polarity within each segment [8,9], and genes whose pattern of expression along the length of the body creates a distinct gene code for each segment (this group includes the homeotic genes).

Segmented insects such as the fruit-fly may seem remote from mouse or man, so it has been quite extraordinary during the past 5 years or so to discover that not only do vertebrate embryos use the same kind of interacting cascades of gene expression as insects, but they use virtually the same genes, which have been highly conserved during evolution [10-12]. This close relationship between ourselves and fruit-flies is easier to understand when the structure of the early mammalian embryo is compared with that of the fly embryo: both have a segmented morphological organisation, and segmented patterns of gene expression corresponding between the two embryo types at comparable levels of the head and trunk.

Retinoic Acid Receptors and Retinoid Binding Proteins in Embryos

Retinoids are involved in all aspects of embryogenesis, i.e., growth, differentiation and morphogenesis. It is therefore not possible to make a deliberate decision to study the roles of retinoids in one of these processes. The embryo, or a major part of it, must be taken as a coordinated system in which the roles of retinoids in determining developmental pattern may be elucidated. The two parts of the embryo that are best understood in this context are the early hindbrain and the limb. Ironically I think that this is because retinoids have very little to do with the normal development of these structures, so it has been relatively simple to show that giving retinoids in excess leads to abnormal development.

The molecular signalling pathways for retinoic acid (RA) in embryogenesis are assumed to be the same as those in other contexts. Nuclear retinoic acid receptors, whose natural ligand is all-*trans* retinoic acid, form heterodimers with retinoid X receptors, whose natural ligand is 9-*cis* retinoic acid [13]. The heterodimers bind to retinoic acid response elements (RAREs) on RA-responsive genes, resulting in the initiation or suppression of transcription. Although the RXRs are ubiquitously necessary for RAR activity, their distribution in embryos is not very informative in relation to retinoid function because they also form heterodimers with related hormone receptors. In contrast, RARs are specifically involved with the retinoid signalling pathway, and their distribution in embryos may be a useful indicator of their functional significance. There are 3 RAR subtypes, α, ß and γ, each of which has a number of isoforms (see Zelent, this volume, for further details and references).

Two methods have been used for studying the distribution of RARs in embryos. The first is *in situ* hybridisation, which reveals the localisation of RNA transcripts of a specific gene, i.e., the position within the embryo in which the gene is being expressed. This method has been used for all of the RARs, and for the retinoid binding proteins, for all stages of mouse prenatal development [14-19]. The second method is the production of transgenic mice, in which the promoter of the gene of choice is linked with the *LacZ* vector from *E.coli* and injected into fertilised eggs. This is essentially a method for labelling the promoter, whose sites of activity can then be localised in embryos at later stages. This method has been used for RAR-ß2 [20].

In addition to the RARs, 3 cytoplasmic retinoid binding proteins are present in embryos. These are cellular retinol binding protein type I (CRBP I) and cellular retinoic acid binding proteins type I and II (CRABP I and CRABP II). (CRBP II is not present during embryogenesis, being first expressed in the differentiated fetal liver and gut.) The function of CRABP II is not understood, and its distribution patterns in embryos [18] do not provide any clues. Compared with CRABP I, it has a lower affinity for retinoic acid, with a dissociation constant 15 times higher (Kd 4.2 nM for CRABP I [21], Kd 65 nM for CRABP II [22]). Unlike CRABP I it is RA-inducible [23]; its patterns of expression show some overlaps with those of RAR-ß and CRBP I, which are also RA-inducible. Its high dissociation constant is compatible with the possibility that it binds RA on a temporary basis, so it could be involved in the transfer of cytoplasmic RA to the nucleus in some cells. Studies on retinoid metabolism indicate that CRBP I binds retinol and facilitates its interactions with dehydrogenases in the synthesis of retinoic acid; in contrast, CRABP I mediates the degradation of RA to inactive metabolites [24]. In embryos, CRBP I is present in the yolk sac placenta [16], where it is well placed to bind retinol from maternal blood for transfer to the embryo. Within the embryo, CRBP I is not ubiquitous but is present in specific cell populations, suggesting that RA synthesis is localised to the tissues in which it is used, with some short-range movement to adjacent tissues. Overlaps between CRBP I and CRABP I are very rare, and the data from their distribution in embryos at all stages of development, and of the effects of RA excess, suggest that CRABP I-mediated degradation of RA is the mechanism whereby nuclear access of RA is limited or prevented. The relationship between retinoids, their cytoplasmic binding proteins, and nuclear receptors, is presented in simplified form in Figure 2, and their distribution in day 9 mouse embryos is shown in Figure 3.

Although each of the RAR subtypes has a specific spatiotemporal distribution in embryos, we know very little about their individual functions. Construction of "knockout" mice that lack the RAR-α or RAR-ß2 genes [25,26] have been disappointingly uninformative, and it is clear that there is a lot of plasticity (functional redundancy) in the RAR system. The phenotype of RAR-γ null mutants shows features similar to the effects of vitamin A deficiency [27]. Correlations of RAR expression patterns with embryo morphology suggest that in normal embryos there may be some specific func-

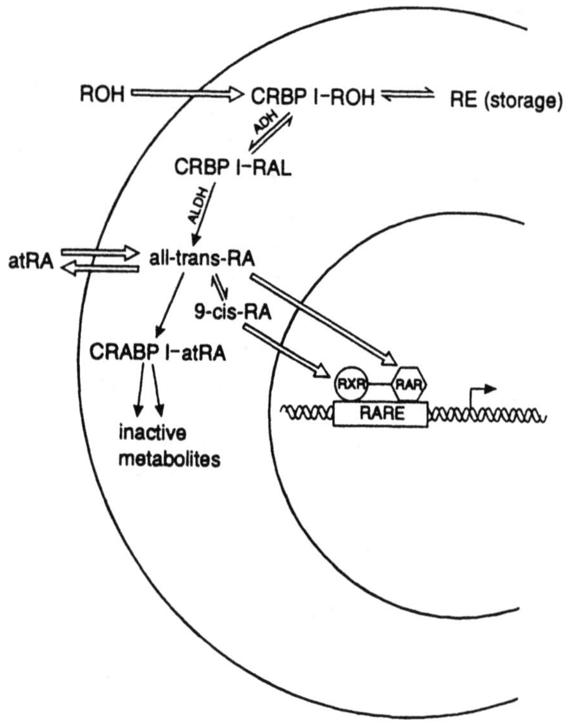

Fig. 2. Summary of retinoid metabolism and binding to cytoplasmic binding proteins and nuclear receptors as described in the text. Open arrows indicate movement of retinoids from extracellular to cytoplasmic and cytoplasmic to nuclear compartments. The source of RA may be intracellular (in which case it may also be exported) if CRBP I is present, or it may enter the cell from an adjacent source. The pathway involving RAR-mediated inhibition of cJun/cFos heterodimer binding to the AP-1 site [46] is not shown.

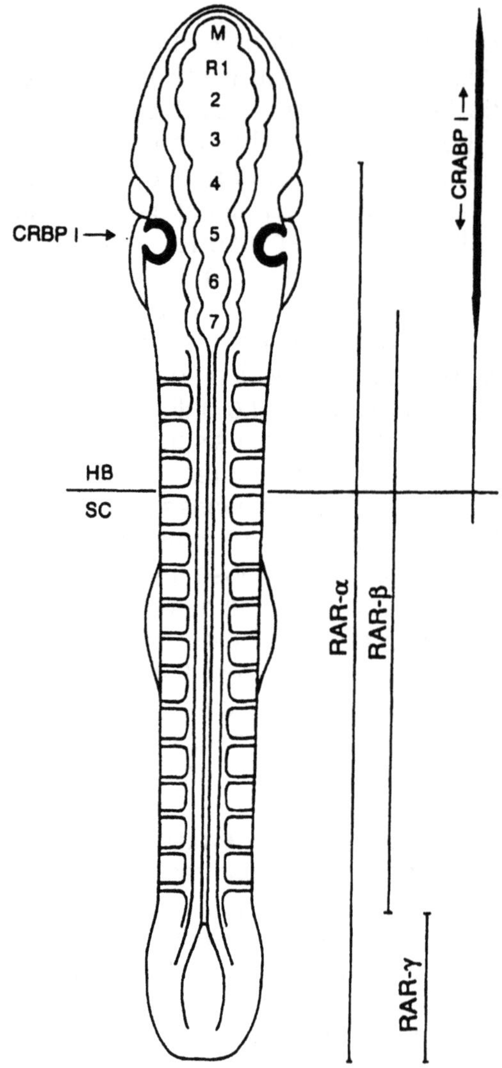

Fig. 3. Diagrammatic representation of a day 9 mouse embryo, dorsal view. The horizontal line demarcates the hindbrain/spinal cord junction (HB/SC). The localisation of RAR and CRABP I transcripts in the neural epithelium is indicated by vertical bars to the right of the embryo. CRABP I expression shows a changing pattern during neurulation, but is generally high in the rostral hindbrain. CRBP I levels are low in the neural epithelium, but high in the otic pit (the precursor of the inner ear, indicated in black). CRABP II expression also shows a changing pattern during neurulation [18] (not shown). RAR-ß and RAR-γ show a reciprocal pattern in the closed and open parts of the spinal cord until the neural tube closes. Based on data from [16]

tions, particularly for RAR-ß and RAR-γ. These two genes show a reciprocal pattern of expression in the closed and open regions of the trunk neural tube (future spinal cord), suggesting roles in neural tube closure and the onset of neural differentiation [16] (Fig. 3). RAR-γ is expressed in the developing digits (precartilage and cartilage tissues) of the hand, whereas RAR-ß is expressed between the developing digits, and it has been suggested that it plays a role in the programme of apoptosis as the digits separate [14]. However, detailed comparison between the patterns of interdigital cell death and of RAR-ß expression reveals that the two sites are mutually exclusive, and that RAR-ß promoter activity coincides with areas where muscle and connective tissue components are differentiating between the skeletal elements [18] (Fig. 4). It may be that interdigital expression of RAR-ß, which is RA-inducible, simply reflects the fact that RA levels are higher between the digits than within them. This pattern of high and low levels of RA within the handplate would enable cartilage to differentiate where RA levels are low, but would inhibit chondrogenesis where RA levels are higher. The inhibitory effects of RA on cartilage differentiation are well known [28-30].

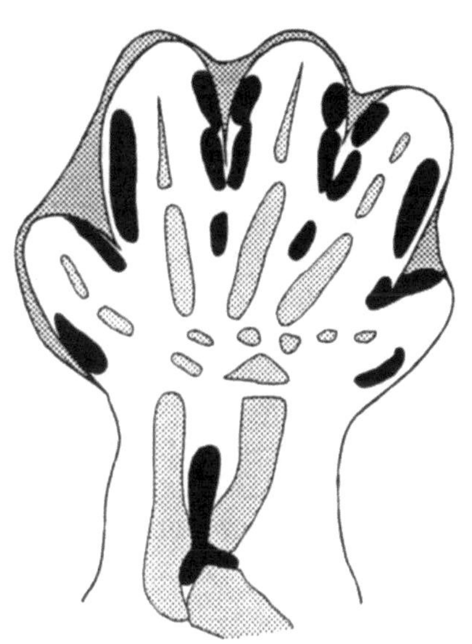

Fig. 4. Embryonic mouse forelimb, day 13.5. Outer stippled areas (mainly between the digits) show areas of cell death; black represents areas of RAR-ß2 promoter activity; inner areas of pale stipple show cartilage. None of these components overlap. Compound drawing compiled from separate preparations illustrated in Figure 9 from [19]

Effects of Altered Retinoid Levels on Embryonic Development

Retinoid levels that are outside the normal physiological range cause abnormal development (Fig. 5). Different patterns of abnormality are caused by vitamin A deficiency and retinoid excess, suggesting that different developmental processes are disrupted. The expression patterns of the two retinoid binding proteins, CRBP I and CRABP I, provide some useful insights into the molecular basis of developmental disruption caused by retinoid excess and deficiency states.

Retinoid Excess

Administration of retinoic acid to a pregnant mouse or rat results in a short pulse of raised RA levels within the embryos, with a peak around 2 hours after maternal dosing, followed by a rapid fall to undetectable levels [31-33]. Because the raised RA level is transitory, the nature of the developmental effect depends on the precise stage of development the embryo has achieved at the time [34]. Changes in the pattern of gene expression triggered by this transitory rise have permanent effects on morphogenesis. Some of the effects on gene expression are also much longer lasting than might be expected: when the RA levels fall, genes that have been upregulated by the raised RA levels may continue to be expressed at an abnormally high level for several days, which is a very long period in developmental time as far as the mouse embryo is concerned. For instance, the induction effect of RA on RAR-ß2 promoter activity in mouse embryos can be seen for at least 48 hours after embryonic exposure to raised RA on day 10 of development [35]. Similarly, effects on the level and pattern of expression of two transforming growth factors, TGF-ß1 and TGF-ß2, are evident more than 24 hours after exposure to RA [36].

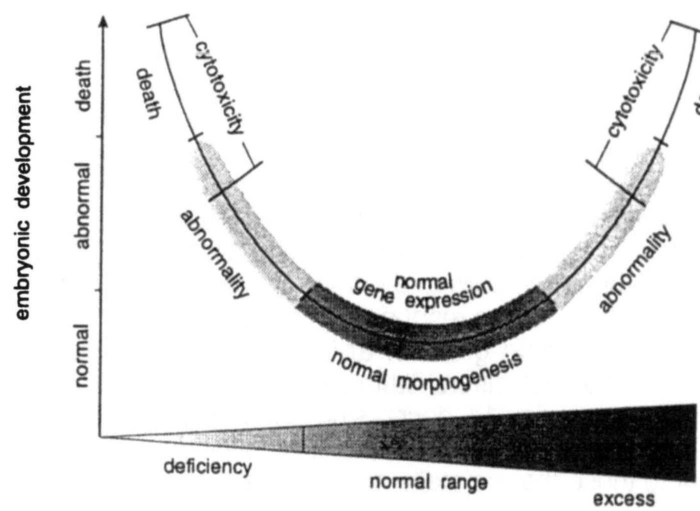

Fig. 5. Summary of the relationship between retinoid deficiency or excess, gene expression and morphogenesis

In general, embryonic tissues in which raised retinoic acid levels cause alteration of the developmental programme are those that show high levels of CRABP I expression. One example is part of the early hindbrain, together with its premigratory neural crest cells, which after migration play a major role in formation of the face. Exposure of both rodent [37] and human [38] embryos to excess retinoic acid at the time of hindbrain neuroepithelium formation results in major abnormality of the face, ears and rostral hindbrain (cerebellum and pons). The first sign of abnormality is a shortened preotic hindbrain and fused or reduced first and second pharyngeal arches [37]. The cerebellum and pons are formed from the preotic hindbrain, and neural crest cells forming the lower jaw and ear ossicles migrate from this region. Another example is the limb. Exposure of mouse embryos to high levels of RA at the early limb bud stage results in abnormalities of the limb skeleton [39]. CRABP I (and II) are present throughout the limb bud at this stage, whereas CRBP I and RAR-ß are excluded except for a small proximal region [18].

My interpretation of these results is that in the early hindbrain and limb buds, high CRABP I levels normally prevent RA from gaining access to the nuclear receptors, so that RA does not play a role in the normal developmental programme. When RA levels are raised sufficiently to overcome the capacity of CRABP I to bind and degrade it, some RA reaches the nucleus, where its activation of the retinoid receptors causes transcription of genes that are not normally transcribed in that region at that time, thus altering the developmental programme.

CRABP I may also modulate the normal differentiation pathway of a given tissue. In the developing mouse cochlea, the sensory epithelium begins to differentiate on day 14, so that at birth there is a single row of inner hair cells and three rows of outer hair cells along the length of the cochlea. The cochlear sensory epithelium differentiates normally in culture, so is quite accessible for experimental manipulation. If low levels of RA are added to the culture medium, 2 rows of inner hair cells and 6 rows of outer hair cells are formed; the response is concentration dependent, being greatest at 5×10^{-8} M RA [40]. The hair cell differentiation response to RA is maximal on day 14, decreasing exponentially thereafter. It indicates that epithelial cells adjacent to those that normally differentiate to form hair cells have the ability to differentiate in the same way, but are not normally stimulated to do so. The timing of the decline in the RA-induced differentiation response coincides with the timing of the synthesis of CRABP I, which first appears at low levels in the cochlea on day 14, reaching high levels by day 16. RA is present in the normal cochlea during the period of hair cell differentiation, and I suggest that the normal function of CRABP I in this context involves limitation of the differentiation response to RA. It would be interesting to discover whether inactivation of CRABP I would result in an increase in the number of hair cells without any addition of RA.

Retinoid Deficiency

In contrast to CRABP I, the pattern of CRBP I expression coincides with tissues that are vulnerable to the effects of vitamin A deficiency. One of these is the lung, in which the respiratory epithelium fails to differentiate normally in conditions of severe vitamin A deficiency, so that the alveoli may fail to expand after birth. This effect has been shown in congenitally vitamin A-deficient mouse embryos (N. Sokolova and G. Morriss-Kay, unpublished observations), and it has also been reported that vitamin A deficiency is a common feature of premature babies showing respiratory distress syndrome [41]. Lung development is an example of morphogenesis involving epithelial-mesenchymal interaction: lung mesenchyme is essential for induction of repeated branching of the initially simple lung buds [42]. When branching is complete, the terminal sac epithelium differentiates to form alveoli, with type 1 pneumocytes (which form the respiratory exchange membrane) and type 2 pneumocytes (the surfactant-secreting cells). Ciliated cells, mucus-secreting cells, and a range of minority cell types differentiate from the epithelium of the bronchioles. These differentiation events require adequate levels of retinol to be available to the developing lung from early branching morphogenesis stages onwards. At present there is no certain method of identifying sites of retinoic acid synthesis at the cellular level, but the presence of CRBP I in a specific tissue at least indicates that the machinery for RA synthesis is present. In the embryonic lung, CRBP I is present in the mesenchyme, but not in the

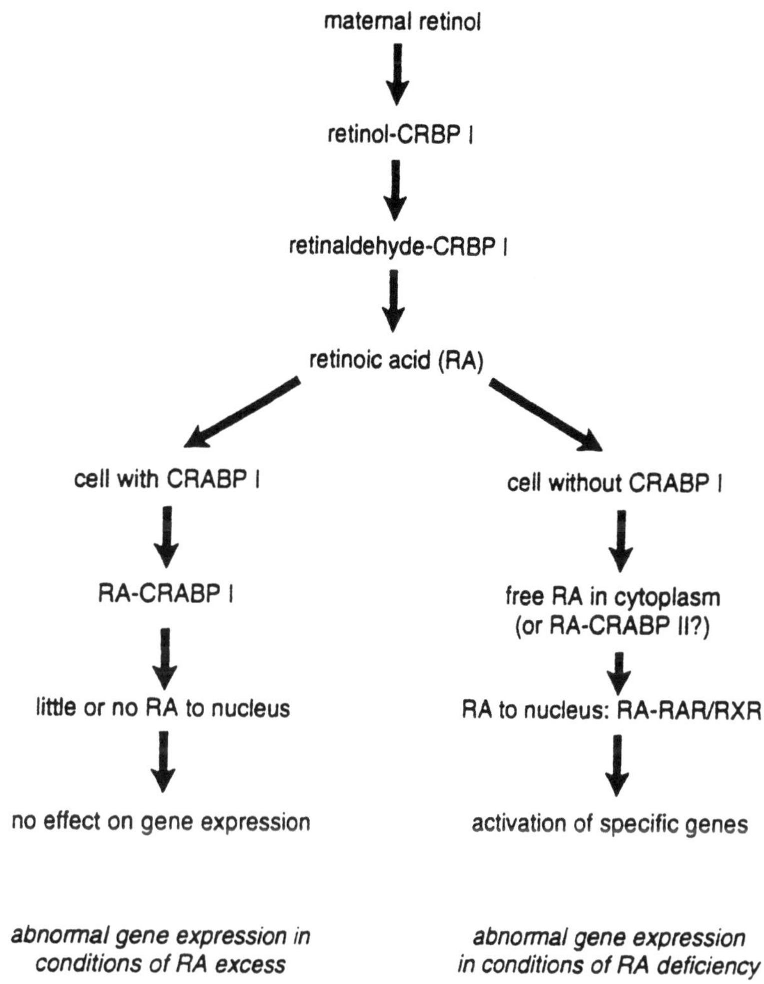

Fig. 6. Summary of the developmental significance of tissue-specific localisation of cytoplasmic retinoid-binding proteins in embryonic tissues

epithelium [15], yet it is the epithelial alveoli that fail to develop normally when retinol is unavailable. At day 14.5 RAR-ß transcripts are present in the differentiating bronchiolar epithelium but not in the terminal sacs, which are still actively branching, suggesting that access of RA to the epithelium may be restricted to the differentiating regions.

My interpretation of the significance of CRBP I and CRABP I in the normal embryonic programme of gene expression, and in conditions of retinoic acid excess or deficiency, is summarised in Figure 6.

Differential Control of Retinoid Levels in Diverging Cell Lineages

Differential localization of CRBP I and CRABP I may enable differential levels of availability of RA to the cell nucleus to be generated and maintained between different tissues, as described above; the same mechanism may act within a tissue, enabling two different pathways of differentiation to emerge from a single cell population. The developing olfactory epithelium is a good candidate for a cell population in which this fine control of differential RA levels enables different programmes of gene expression to be followed within a tissue. At first the olfactory epithelium (olfactory placode) consists of a single cell type, and CRBP I transcripts are present in both the epithelium and the adjacent mesenchyme [15]. CRBP I transcripts are subsequently lost from the epithelium (but remain in the mesenchyme) when a subpopulation of the epithelial cells, positioned in the middle of the thickness of the epithelium, begin to differentiate as olfactory receptor cells. Further cell lineage divergence occurs when the apical layer epithelial cells cease to be stem cells and begin to differentiate as supporting cells [43]. At this stage (Fig. 7) differential expression of RAR-ß and CRABP I within the epithelium indicates that RA levels are higher in the apical cells (supporting cell line), in which

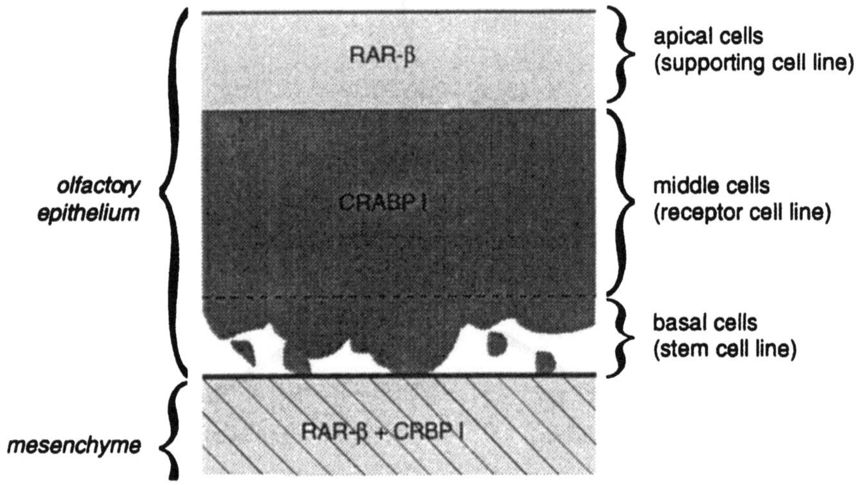

Fig. 7. Diagrammatic summary of RA-related gene expression in the olfactory epithelium and underlying mesenchyme, in relation to the 3 cell populations within the epithelium. Data from [15]

the RA-inducible gene RAR-ß is expressed, than in the developing receptor cells, in which the RA-degrading binding protein CRABP I is expressed. Patchy CRABP I expression is also detected in the stem cell population. CRBP I is restricted to the mesenchyme, which is therefore likely to be the site of synthesis of the RA that enters the epithelial cells. These observations suggest that fine control of RA levels, by means of differential synthesis of the binding proteins that mediate synthesis and degradation of RA, can occur in different cell lineages within the same tissue. Differential RA levels may play an important role in the emergence or maintenance of those separate lineages, by initiating separate gene expression pathways. Restriction of the machinery for RA synthesis to the mesenchyme, and expression of an RA-inducible gene in the apical epithelial cell population, gives some indication of the distances that secreted RA can traverse (approximately 100 μm in this example).

Binding Protein Synthesis and Retinoid Levels

I have emphasized the role of binding proteins in controlling the retinoid signalling pathway in different embryonic tissues as an important factor in the generation of tissue diversity. I will end with a short postscript describing two experimental examples indicating that levels of binding protein expression are themselves affected by retinoid levels.

1) As discussed above, normal lung development fails if retinoid levels are deficient. Vitamin A deficiency can be mimicked in culture by the use of retinol-free serum; in these conditions, CRBP I levels are raised, in comparison with lungs cultured in medium containing physiological levels of retinol (N. Sokolova and G. Morriss-Kay, unpublished observations). CRBP I is a retinoic acid-inducible gene, so this response is the opposite of what would be expected from the molecular data.

2) In the day 8.0 mouse embryo, CRABP I expression is confined to the embryonic midbrain and hindbrain neuroepithelium, and soon afterwards can be seen in the migrating cranial neural crest cells. Following exposure to RA excess on day 8.0, *in situ* hybridisation shows CRABP I transcripts in a number of ectopic sites, including the forebrain and the trunk [43]. Thus part of the response of embryos to RA excess is upregulation of CRABP I. CRABP I is not known to be an RA-inducible gene, so again, this is not the response one would predict.

In both of these examples, it is tempting to say that the embryo is responding protectively: deficiency of retinoic acid leads to generation of more of the machinery for its synthesis; excess retinoic acid leads to synthesis of more of the means to protect against its effects. These interpretations are speculative and teleological, but they may contain a grain of truth. The second example has a parallel in a clinical therapeutic observation: in acute promyelocytic leukaemia, the abnormal promyelocytes can be stimulated to differentiate by RA, but they eventually become refractory to this treatment; the onset of resistance is correlated with the appearance of CRABP I in the bone marrow

[44]. There may be many other ways in which study of the retinoid signalling pathway in embryonic tissues can provide insight into the therapeutic potential of retinoids in relation to cancer.

Acknowledgements

Work from my laboratory described in this chapter was supported by the Human Frontier Science Program and by Hoffmann-La Roche.

REFERENCES

1 Bernfield M, Banerjee SD, Koda J, Rapraeger AC: Remodeling of the basement membrane as a mechanism of morphogenetic tissue interaction. In: Trelstad RL (ed) The Role of Extracellular Matrix in Development. Alan R Liss, Inc, New York 1984 pp 545-572

2 Nakanishi Y, Morita T, Nogawa M: Cell proliferation is not required for the initiation of early cleft formation in mouse embryonic submandibular epithelium in vitro. Development 1987 (99):429-437

3 Morriss-Kay GM: Growth and development of pattern in the cranial neural epithelium of rat embryos during neurulation. J Embryol Exp Morph 1981 (65 suppl):225-241

4 Conlon RA and Rossant J: Exogenous retinoic acid rapidly induces anterior ectopic expression of murine *Hox-2* genes in vivo. Development 1992 (116): 357-368

5 Langman J, Guerrant RL, Freemen BG: Behavior of neuroepithelial cells during closure of the neural tube. J Comp Neurol (127):399-412

6 Morriss-Kay G and Mahmood R: Morphogenesis-related changes in extracellular matrix induced by retinoic acid. In: Morriss-Kay GM (ed) Retinoids in Normal Development and Teratogenesis. Oxford University Press, Oxford 1992 pp 165-180

7 Tuckett F, Morriss-Kay GM: A role for heparan sulphate proteoglycan in the rat embryo: effects of heparitinase treatment during early organogenesis. Anat Embryol 1989 (180):393-400

8 Nüsslein-Volhard C and Wieschaus E: Mutations affecting segment number and polarity in *Drosophila*. Nature 1980 (287):795-801

9 Ingham PW:Localised *hedgehog* activity controls spatially restricted transcription of *wingless* in the *Drosophila* embryo. Nature 1993 (366):560-562

10 Duboule D and Dollé P: The structural and functional organization of the murine HOX gene family resembles that of *Drosophila* homeotic genes. EMBO J 1989 (8):1497-1505

11 Graham A, Papalopulu N, Krumlauf R: The murine and *Drosophila* homeobox clusters have common features of organisation and expression. Cell 1989 (57):367-378

12 Ingham P: *Hedgehog* points the way. Current Biology 1994 (4):347-350

13 Mangelsdorf DJ, Umesono K, Evans RM: The retinoid receptors. In: Sporn MB, Roberts AB, Goodman DS (eds) The Retinoids. Raven Press Ltd, New York 1994 pp 319-349

14 Dollé P, Ruberte E, Kastner P, Petkovich M, Stoner CM, Gudas LJ, Chambon P: Differential expression of the genes encoding the retinoic acid receptors α, ß, γ and CRABP in the developing limbs of the mouse. Nature 1989 (342):702-705

15 Dollé P, Ruberte E, Leroy P, Morriss-Kay G, Chambon P: Retinoic acid receptors and cellular binding proteins I. A systematic study of their differential pattern of transcription during mouse organogenesis. Development 1990 (110):1133-1151

16 Ruberte E, Dollé P, Chambon P, Morriss-Kay G: Retinoic acid receptors and cellular binding proteins II. Their differential pattern of transcription during early morphogenesis in mouse embryos. Development 1991 (111):45-60

17 Ruberte E, Nakshatri H, Kastner P, Chambon P: Retinoic acid receptors and binding proteins in mouse limb development. In: GM Morriss-Kay (ed) Retinoids in Normal Development and Teratogenesis. Oxford University Press, Oxford 1992 pp 99-111

18 Ruberte E, Friederich V, Morriss-Kay G, Chambon P: Differential distribution patterns of CRABP I and CRABP II transcripts during mouse embryogenesis. Development 1992 (115):973-987

19 Ruberte E, Friederich V, Chambon P, Morriss-Kay G: Retinoic acid receptors and cellular retinoid binding proteins III. Their differential transcript distribution during mouse nervous system development. Development 1993 (118):267-282

20 Mendelsohn C, Ruberte E, LeMeur M, Morriss-Kay G, Chambon P: Developmental analysis of the retinoic acid inducible RAR-ß2 promoter in transgenic animals. Development 1991 (113):723-734

21 Ong D and Chytil F: Cellular retinoic acid binding protein from rat testis. J Biol Chem 1978 (253):4551-4554

22 Bailey JS and Siu CH: Purification and partial characterization of a novel binding protein for retinoic acid from neonatal rat. J Biol Chem 1988 (263): 9326-9332

23 Giguère V, Lyn S, Yip P, Siu CH, Amin S: Molecular cloning of cDNA encoding a second cellular retinoic acid-binding protein. Proc Natl Acad Sci USA 1990 (87):6233-6237

24 Napoli JL: Biosynthesis and metabolism of retinoic acid: roles of CRBP and CRABP in retinoic acid homeostasis. J Nutr 1993 (123):362-366

25 Lufkin T, Mark M, Hart CP et al: High postnatal lethality and testis degeneration in retinoic acid receptor α mutant mice. Proc Natl Acad Sci USA 1993 (90):7225-7229

26 Lohnes D, Kastner p, Dierich A, Mark M, LeMeur M, Chambon P: Function of retinoic acid receptor γ in the mouse. Cell 1993 (73):643-658

27 Mendelsohn C, Mark M, Dollé P et al: Retinoic acid receptor ß2 (RARß2) null mutant mice appear normal. Developmental Biology 1994 (in press)

28 Fell HB and Mellanby E: The effect of hypervitaminosis A on embryonic limb-bones cultivated in vitro. J Physiol 1952 (116):320-349

29 Shapiro SS and Mott DJ: Modulation of glycosaminoglycan biosynthesis by retinoids. Ann NY Acad Sci 1981 (359):306-321

30 Kistler A: Hypervitaminosis A: side-effects of retinoids. Biochem Soc Trans 1986 (14):936-939

31 Creech Kraft J, Löfberg B, Chahoud I, Bochert G, Nau H: Teratogenicity and placental transfer of all-*trans*, 13-*cis*, 4-oxo-all-*trans*, and 4-oxo-13-*cis*-retinoic acid after a low oral dose during organogenesis in mice. Toxicol Appl Pharmacol 1989 (100):162-176

32 Satre MA and Kochhar DM: Elevations in the endogenous levels of the putative morphogen retinoic acid in embryonic mouse limb buds associated with limb dysmorphogenesis. Devel Biol 1989 (133):529-536

33 Ward SJ and Morriss-Kay GM: Distribution of all-

trans-, 13-*cis*- and 9-*cis*-retinoic acid to whole rat embryos and maternal serum following oral administration of a teratogenic dose of all-*trans*-retinoic acid. Pharmacol Toxicol 1994 (in press)
34 Wood H, Pall G, Morriss-Kay G: Exposure to retinoic acid before or after the onset of somitogenesis reveals separate effects on rhombomeric segmentation and 3' *HoxB* gene expression domains. Development 1994 (120):2279-2285
35 Ward S: The roles of retinoic acid in normal and abnormal mammalian limb development. Ph.D. thesis, University of Oxford, 1994
36 Mahmood R, Flanders KC, Morriss-Kay GM: Interactions between retinoids and TGF-ßs in mouse morphogenesis. Development 1992 (115):67-74
37 Morriss-Kay GM: Retinoic acid and craniofacial development: molecules and morphogenesis. BioEssays 1993 (15):9-15
38 Lammer EJ, Chen DT, Hoar RM et al: Retinoic acid embryopathy. New Engl J Med 1985 (313):837-841
39 Kochhar DM: Limb development in mouse embryos. I. Analysis of teratogenic effects of retinoic acid. Teratology 1973 (11):289-298
40 Kelley MW, Xu XM, Wagner MA, Warchol ME, Corwin JT: The developing organ of Corti contains retinoic acid and forms supernumerary hair cells in response to exogenous retinoic acid in culture. Development 1993 (119):1041-1053
41 Shenai JP, Kennedy KA, Chytil F, Stahlman MT: Clinical trial of vitamin A supplementation in infants susceptible to bronchopulmonary dysplasia. J Pediatr 1987 (111):269-277
42 Wessels NK: Mammalian lung development: interactions in formation and morphogenesis of tracheal buds. J Exp Zool 1970 (175):455-466
43 Cuschieri A and Bannister LH: The development of the olfactory mucosa in the mouse: light microscopy. J Anat 1975 (119):277-286
44 Pall GS: The effects of excess retinoic acid on the expression of retinoid signalling pathway genes and morphogenesis in mouse embryos. M.Sc. thesis, University of Oxford, 1994
45 Cornic M, Delva L, Guidez F, Balitrand N, Degos L, Chomienne C: Induction of retinoic acid-binding protein in normal and malignant myeloid cells by retinoic acid in acute promyelocytic leukemia patients. Cancer Res 1992 (52):3329-3334
46 Yang-Yen H-F, Zhang X-K, Graupner G, Tzukerman M, Sakamoto B, Karin M, Pfahl M: Antagonism between retinoic acid receptors and AP-1: Implications for tumor promotion and inflammation. New Biologist 1991 (3):1206-1220

Clinical Pharmacology of the Retinoids

Ugo Pastorino [1], Raymond P. Warrell, Jr [2] and Franca Formelli [3]

1 Department of Thoracic Surgery, Istituto Nazionale Tumori, Via Venezian 1, 20133 Milan, Italy
2 Department of Medicine, Memorial Sloan-Kettering Cancer Center, 1275 York Avenue, New York, NY 10021, U.S.A.
3 Department of Experimental Oncology B, Istituto Nazionale Tumori, Via Venezian 1, 20133 Milan, Italy

Positive results achieved with retinoids in the chemoprevention of epithelial cancer as well as in the treatment of acute promyelocytic leukaemia and squamous cancers of the skin and cervix have stimulated interest in the pharmacological aspects of these substances. The use of retinoids in clinical oncology and particularly in chemoprevention poses specific problems of tolerability, whether the agents are used singly or in combination with other anticancer drugs. A particular characteristic of cancer chemoprevention is the requirement for precise assessment of metabolic and toxicologic profiles related to long-term administration.

The term "retinoids" comprises a highly heterogeneous group of substances (Fig. 1), with peculiar properties in terms of absorption, metabolism, pharmacokinetics, bioavailability and toxicity. As an example, Table 1 shows the plasma elimination half-lives of the different retinoids discussed in this chapter (all-*trans* RA, 13-*cis* RA, 4-HPR) and of other retinoids employed mainly in dermatology (etretinate, acitretin). The following sections deal with the pharmacological characteristics of the major retinoids which have been used to date in clinical oncology.

Retinol

Natural vitamin A (all-*trans* retinol, retinal, and retinyl esters) is essential for vision, reproduction, and maintenance of differentiated epithelia and mucus secretion in humans and higher animals [6]. *Trans* retinoic acid shares only a part of these functions, being unable to support vision and reproduction; therefore animals maintained on retinoic acid as the only source of vitamin A are both blind and sterile. Retinol is stored in the liver in large amounts (over 90% of the total supply), which normally exceed the physiological requirement for 1 year. Vitamin A is released in the plasma and transported bound to a specific retinol-binding protein (RBP). The process of mobilisation is mainly controlled by the liver, although recycling from peripheral tissues and extravascular spaces may also be relevant, according to recent studies [7]. Retinol plasma levels are maintained generally stable except in extreme conditions, such as chronic dietary deficiency or high-dose supplementation.

Table 1. Plasma elimination half-lives of various retinoids administered orally to humans

	Half-life in hours	Reference	
All-*trans* retinoic acid	0.8 ± 0,1	Muindi, 1992	[1]
13-*cis* retinoic acid	10 (6.7-36.5)	Brazzell, 1983	[2]
Fenretinide (4-HPR)	27 ± 4	Formelli, 1993	[3]
Etretinate	2500*	Massarella, 1985	[4]
Acitretin	50 (36-96)	Wiegand, 1993	[5]

* over 120 days

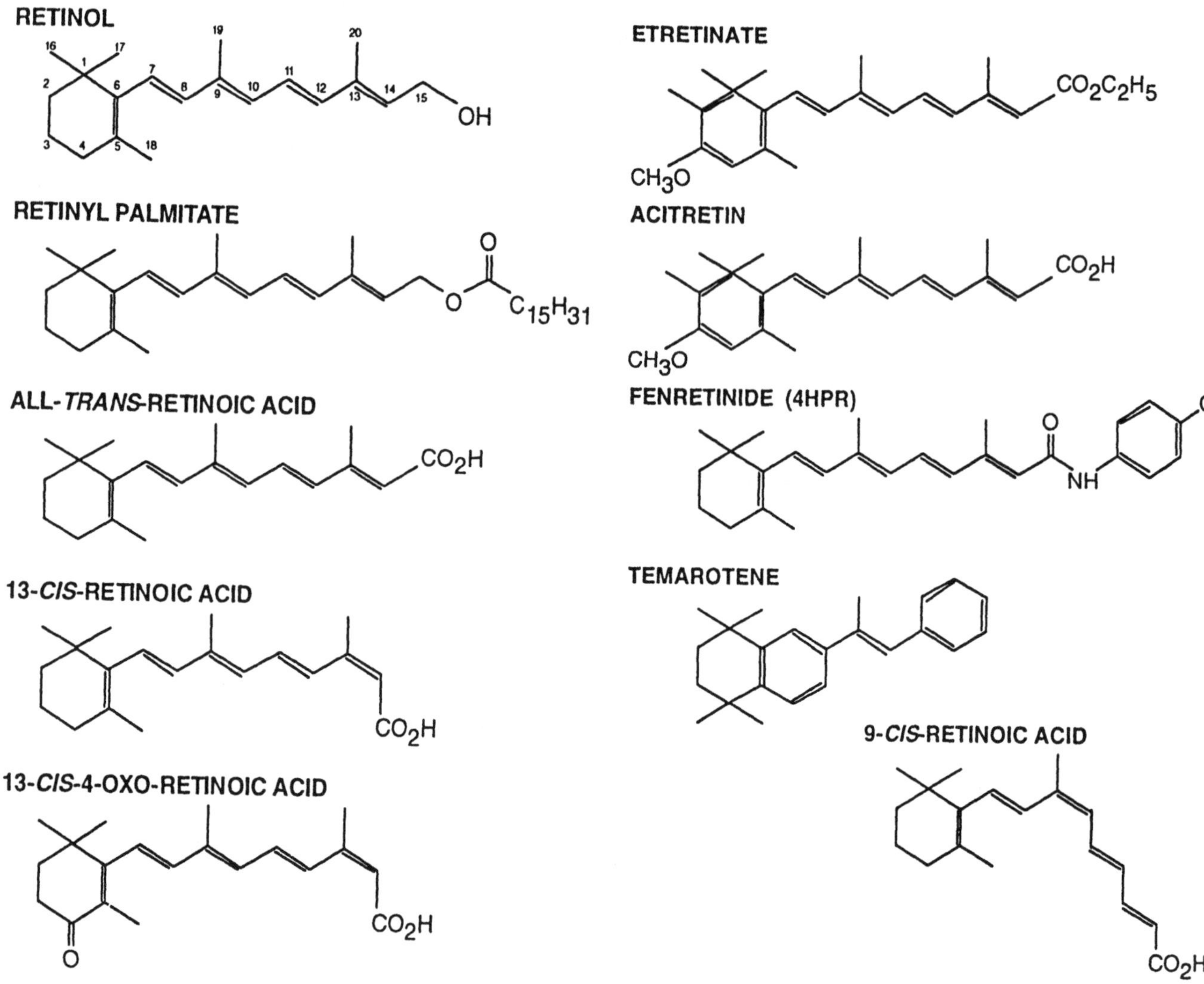

Fig. 1. Chemical structure of different retinoids

The Pharmacokinetics of Oral Supplementation

The pharmacokinetics of orally administered retinol are dominated by strong homeostatic mechanisms, and a number of studies using low-dose vitamin A have failed to show any significant change in plasma retinol levels. A randomised double-blind trial including 376 volunteers has shown that oral administration of retinyl palmitate at moderate doses (10,000 to 36,000 IU daily) induces a slight but significant increase in basal retinol levels, in the order of 2% for every 10,000 IU [8]. In a pilot study involving cancer patients higher doses of oral retinol (up to 200,000 IU/m^2 daily) produced a rapid increase in retinyl palmitate, with a mean time to peak plasma concentrations of nearly 4 hours and an initial phase half-life of 2 hours (Fig. 2) [9]. However, the plasma retinol concentration increased only in patients with low initial levels. The plasma half-life of retinyl palmitate, when retinol was given at a daily dose of 25,000 IU, ranged between 15 and 22 hours [10]. In the experience gathered at the Istituto Nazionale Tumori, based on 307 patients randomised to receive retinyl palmitate or no treatment (control), a daily dose of 300,000 IU was associated with a significant increase in the average values of plasma retinol and retinol-binding protein (greater than 30% and 60%, respectively) after 12 months of treatment [11].

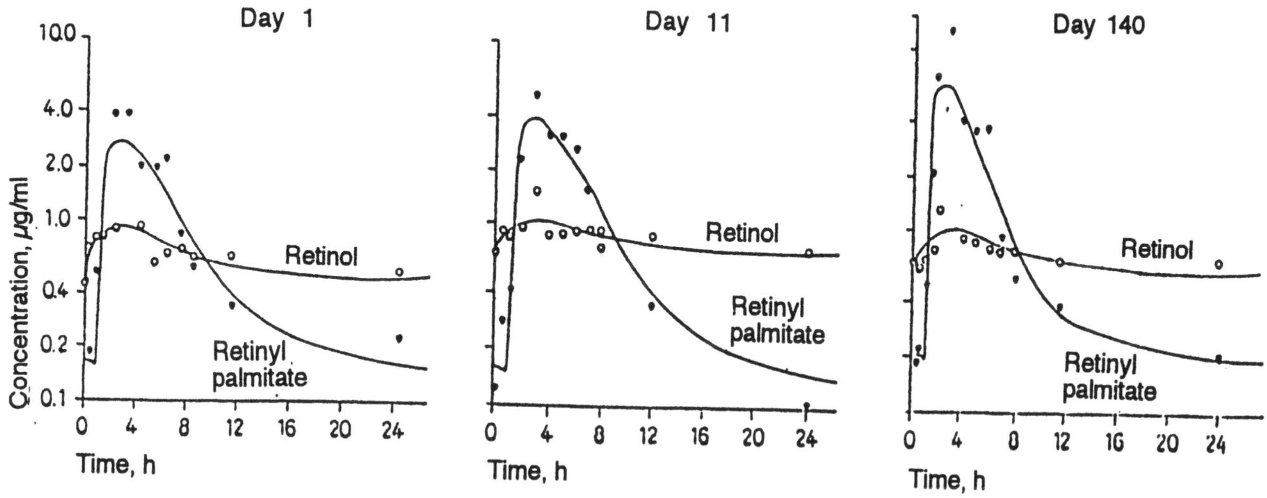

Fig. 2. Serial computer-plotted plasma concentration/time curves for a single patient receiving oral daily retinol, 100,000 U/m2 day. Reproduced with permission from [9]

Physiological Aspects of Retinol Bioavailability

Although it has never been properly evaluated, the intestinal absorption rate in humans is commonly estimated to be 50% to 60% of the total dietary retinol. However, several factors may influence the pharmacology of oral vitamin A supplementation, including the chemical structure (alcohol, esters) and the type of preparation (oily solution, emulsion). For instance, a retrospective study of human toxicity data estimated that the absorption and storage rate of emulsified retinol may be as high as 80%, compared to only 20% for oily solutions [12].

Chemical and physical properties may also be implicated in the pattern of liver toxicity as well as the bioavailability of the substance in extrahepatic tissues. The difference may be prominent between natural substances such as retinol, which are transported almost entirely as chylomicrons in the general circulation and through the lymphatic system, and retinoic acid which is directly transported to the liver through the portal system [13].

Recent evidence to support the clinical relevance of extrahepatic uptake of chylomicron retinyl esters comes from *in vitro* experiments on HL-60 cells, which demonstrated growth inhibition and differentiation after exposure of leukaemic cells to chylomicron retinyl esters [14].

Effect of Long-Term Administration on Biochemical Parameters

In a prospective randomised trial carried out in Milan on the use of emulsified retinyl palmitate at high doses for a long period of time, no significant effects on liver function nor objective liver toxicity were demonstrated with standard laboratory tests. The average liver enzyme values (serum GOT and GPT) measured every month up to 24 months of treatment, were nearly identical in randomised controls and treated individuals, with only a limited proportion of patients (10-20%) showing serum levels above the normal range in both groups [15]. On the other hand, retinyl palmitate administration caused a remarkable increase in serum triglycerides that reached statistical significance at 12 months of treatment, with average values in excess of 60% compared to baseline levels. Such a significant increase in serum triglycerides was not associated with clinical symptoms or objective signs of cardiovascular damage and spontaneously reverted to normal values soon after treatment completion. Cholesterol levels were much less affected, with the differences in mean values not significant between the two groups. Renal function tests, glucose fasting levels, haemoglobin values, RBC, WBC and lymphocyte counts were all not affected by retinyl palmitate administration. These observations underline

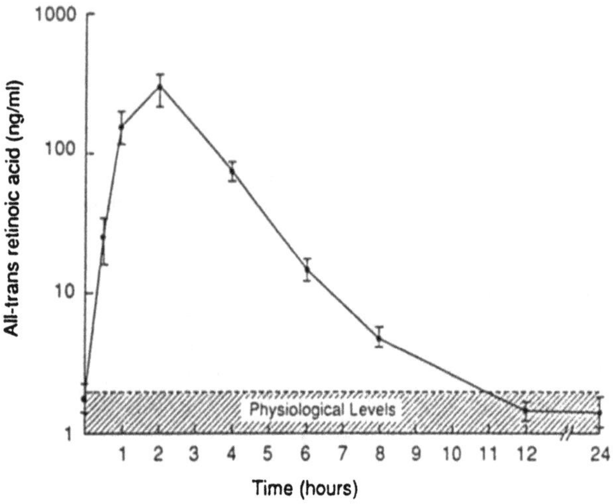

Fig. 3. Plasma concentrations following ingestion of a single dose of all-*trans* RA (45 mg/m^2) on day 1 of treatment. *Points*, means; *bars*, SEM.
Reproduced with permission from [1]

the need for properly controlled studies, possibly in a prospective randomised setting, for an accurate assessment of the side-effects associated with long-term retinol administration.

All-*trans* Retinoic Acid

A large proportion of patients with acute promyelocytic leukaemia (APL) achieve complete remissions after treatment with all-*trans* retinoic acid (RA) [16-24]. Nonetheless, despite the high initial remission rate, the mean duration of remission in patients treated only with all-*trans* RA is relatively brief, averaging 3.5 months in the New York series [23]. Moreover, patients who relapse from a remission induced and maintained by all-*trans* RA are all clinically resistant to further treatment even at escalated doses; in some cases, however, their leukaemic cells appeared to retain sensitivity to the cytodifferentiating actions of the drug *in vitro* [25-27]. These findings suggested that this retinoid might have unique pharmacological properties; this speculation has indeed proven correct.

Pharmacokinetics After Single and Multiple Doses

After administration of a single oral dose, peak plasma concentrations of all-*trans* RA are reached within 1 to 3 hours (Fig. 3) [1,28]. Subsequently, drug levels in plasma decay monoexponentially with a half-life of approximately 40 minutes. These data are in contrast with the plasma half-life of its isomer, 13-*cis* retinoic acid, which approximates 12 to 14 hours. In addition, these data were characterised by considerable interpatient variability. A second surprise was the finding that continuous daily dosing in patients with APL was associated with a progressive decrease in plasma drug concentrations [25]. Later, this finding was shown not to be disease specific and was corroborated by studies in patients with solid tumours. Studies of leukaemic patients who relapsed while on continuous therapy with all-*trans* RA revealed a highly significant decrease in both peak plasma concentrations (Cp_{max}) and in plasma AUC at the time of relapse compared to the first day of treatment. Moreover, a 2-fold increase in the oral dose not only failed to significantly augment the plasma AUC values, but also to recapture the clinical response. These findings suggested that relapse may have been associated with an acquired inability to sustain effective plasma drug concentrations [25]. Although the induced decrease in plasma drug levels was originally observed at the time of leukaemic relapse, more recent studies have shown that this process occurs early during therapy; in many patients, the phenomenon is noted within the first week of dosing [25]. The decrease in Cp_{max} and AUC values was associated with an approximately 10-fold increase in urinary excretion of 4-oxo retinoic acid metabolites. This metabolite exists in urine as a conjugate of glucuronide, as evidenced by the fact that it was only detected after ß-glucuronidase hydrolysis. Very little isomerisation to 13-*cis* retinoic acid was observed in plasma.

Constitutive Variability in Pharmacokinetics of All-trans Retinoic Acid

As noted previously, measurements of the plasma AUC values after an identical oral dose of all-*trans* RA have been highly variable. In a study of patients with non-small cell lung cancer, the median AUC value appeared to be substantially lower than in patients with APL. This observation led to the classification of cancer patients into "normal" or "rapid" catabolizers, based on whether the AUC on the first day of treatment was greater or less than the median value of 250 ng·hr/ml [29]. The importance of this distinction was further highlighted by the observation that patients who were rapid catabolizers had endogenous plasma retinoid levels significantly below those of the normal catabolizers [29].

Putative Mechanism(s) of Accelerated Catabolism

Preclinical studies *in vitro* and in animals suggested that oxidation of all-*trans* RA by cytochrome P450 enzymes was a major pathway of metabolic degradation. In order to assess whether this pathway was clinically important, a broad-spectrum inhibitor of cytochrome P450 oxidases (ketoconazole) was administered on the second and twenty-ninth day of a 1-month treatment period with all-*trans* RA. This study showed that the inducible pattern of accelerated all-*trans* RA catabolism was reliably blocked on day 29 compared to testing on day 28. Moreover, in the group of patients who exhibited the "rapid" catabolic phenotype, the day 2 AUC values were significantly higher than the levels on day 1. By contrast, no differences between days 1 and 2 were observed in patients with the "normal" catabolic phenotype [29]. These findings strongly suggested that both the inducible and the constitutive patterns of accelerated retinoid catabolism were mediated by the same processes and that both could be blocked by an inhibitor of cytochrome P450 oxidases such as ketoconazole. Similar findings were observed by Miller et al. [30] using a different azole inhibitor, liarozole.

The azole compounds mentioned above, however, exert a variety of pharmacological effects in addition to inhibition of P450 oxidases, and one of these actions is inhibition of oxidation by lipid hydroperoxides. Muindi and Young measured the plasma lipid hydroperoxide content in normal volunteers and patients, and they showed that these levels were not different in the volunteers and the patients who exhibited the "normal" catabolic phenotype. However, individuals with the "rapid" catabolic phenotype had significantly higher levels. Moreover, continuous treatment with all-*trans* RA was associated with an increase in plasma lipid peroxide concentrations [31]. Thus, the inhibitory activity of the azole compounds could be due either to their effects on cytochrome P450 oxidases or to an effect on cellular oxidation by lipid hydroperoxides.

Finally, recent studies have suggested that cellular retinoic acid binding proteins (CRABP) were also involved in the catabolic process, perhaps by facilitating the transport of retinoids to the endoplasmic reticulum for subsequent oxidation [32,33]. Chomienne and her colleagues investigated the effects of all-*trans* RA upon mRNA expression of CRABP-II (the predominant protein in myeloid cells) in mononuclear cells from the bone marrow of patients with APL. In these patients serial studies showed that all-*trans* RA treatment was associated with increased expression of CRABP-II [26]. In 3 patients, the time course of this increase was also associated with a relative decrease in the sensitivity of the leukaemic cells to *in vitro* differentiation by all-*trans* RA [26]. Thus, it appears that patients vary considerably in their handling of endogenous retinoids based in part on their endogenous rates of oxidation (whether by the levels of cytochrome P450 oxidase activity or by lipid oxidative cofactors) and possibly on alterations in intracellular expression of retinoic acid binding proteins.

Implications of the Pharmacokinetic Findings for All-trans Retinoic Acid

The above findings have led to speculations regarding the possible mechanisms of native and acquired resistance to the biological actions of all-*trans* retinoic acid, particularly in patients with acute promyelocytic leukaemia [34]. In certain cell lines, acquired resistance in myeloid leukaemia (HL60 and NB4) has arisen via the development of new genetic abnormalities, including point mutations in retinoic acid receptors [35] or altered expression of the mutant PML/RAR-α fusion protein in APL [36]. As yet, however, there is no evidence that such mutations occur to any clinically important extent in human subjects. Evidence against the "mutation hypothesis" is largely circumstantial. Nonetheless, it appears that clinical resistance to all-*trans* RA in APL occurs rapidly and universally, but also that it may be reversible after drug treatment has been discontinued for several months. Each of these features would seem to argue strongly against the development of acquired and heritable retinoic acid receptor mutations in APL cells. These observations have led to the "pharmacological hypothesis" of acquired resistance, namely that continuous exposure to this natural retinoid rapidly induces a variety of metabolic processes (both in the target cell and elsewhere in the body), and that the net effect of these processes is to reduce the effective intranuclear concentrations of the ligand, probably to levels that are inadequate to initiate or sustain cytodifferentiation.

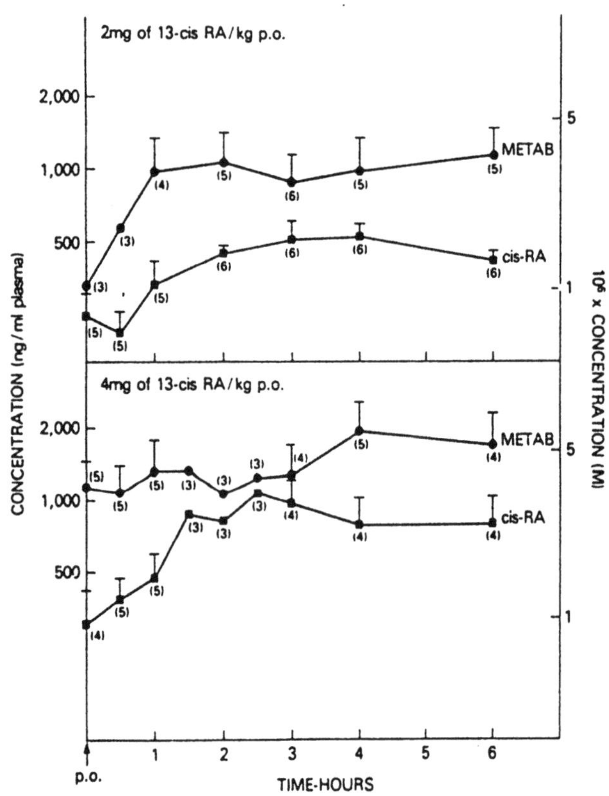

Fig. 4. Plasma 13-*cis* RA and metabolite (METAB) after doses of 2 mg/kg (top) and 4 mg/kg (bottom). *Numbers in parentheses*, number of patients represented at each point. *Points*, mean. *Bars*, S.E. Metabolite concentrations were calculated from the 13-*cis* RA standard curve. The metabolite had the same retention times as did 4-oxo-*trans*-retinoic acid.
Reproduced with permission from [37]

As noted above, several mechanism(s), none of them mutually exclusive, have been proposed whereby this process might occur, and several strategies have been proposed to deal with this problem. The simplest test may be the provision of a large parenteral dose of the retinoid to patients who have developed resistance. However, the optimal strategy may well include the use of a retinoid other than all-*trans* RA that does not induce this process. Several such compounds have been identified and their utility will be explored in the near future.

13-*cis* Retinoic Acid

The increasing interest in the use of synthetic retinoids in oncology is mainly related to the significant results achieved with 13-*cis* retinoic acid (RA) in oral premalignant and malignant diseases. In oral leukoplakia, 13-*cis* RA has induced complete clinical and pathological remissions in a large proportion of patients. In patients treated for a prior head and neck cancer, 13-*cis* RA was effective in preventing the occurrence of second primary tumours. However, two major problems with the use of this drug are the limited tolerability of side-effects with optimal doses, and the recurrence of leukoplakia when the treatment is stopped. In chemoprevention trials very few patients were able to tolerate the dose of 1 mg/kg for periods longer than 6 months. More recent experience with low-dose maintenance (0.5 mg/kg) following full-dose induction appears promising, and new prospective trials have selected a daily dose of 30 mg.

Pharmacokinetics After Single and Multiple Doses

After a single oral dose of 0.5 mg/kg of 13-*cis* RA, the mean peak plasma concentration was 250 ng/ml (range 0-740) and the time to peak plasma concentration 4 hours (range 2-6 hr). After 4 mg/kg p.o. the mean peak plasma concentration was 1160 ng/ml (range 828-1950) and the time to peak plasma concentration 3 hours (range 1.5-6 hr) (Fig. 4) [37]. A marked difference in gastrointestinal absorption was probaby responsible for the great variation in

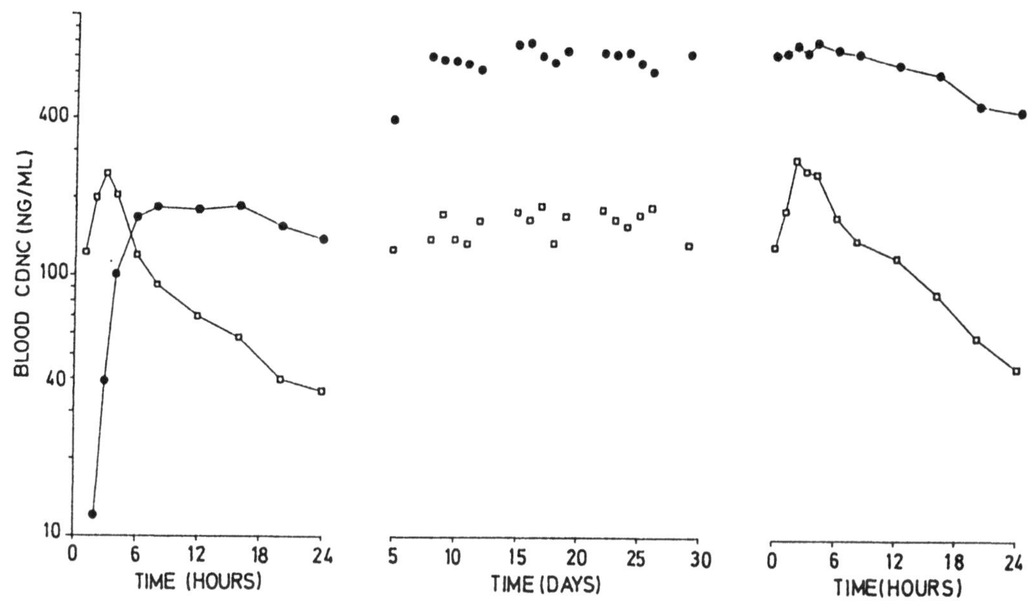

Fig. 5. Isotretinoin (□) and 4-oxo-isotretinoin (●) mean blood concentrations (ng/ml) following multiple-dose administration of isotretinoin to 10 cystic acne patients. The first graph represents the mean concentration-time profiles after the first 80 mg dose of isotretinoin; the second graph is the mean trough concentrations during the 25 days of 40 mg b.i.d. dosing; and the third graph represents the mean concentration-time profiles following an 80 mg single dose administered 12 h after the last 40 mg b.i.d. dose. Reproduced with permission from [2]

peak plasma levels (up to 10-fold) in patients receiving the same dose [9]. A lag time of up to 2 hours was reported prior to the onset of intestinal absorption, as well as marked secondary and tertiary concentration peaks consistent with enterohepatic circulation of 13-*cis* RA [38]. The pharmacokinetics of multiple doses of 13-*cis* RA was tested in 10 patients treated with 40 mg daily for 25 days (Fig. 5) [2]. The peak plasma concentration after 25 days of treatment was similar to that observed after the first dose (310±184 ng/ml versus 262±139 ng/ml), the time to peak plasma levels was 3.1 versus 2.9 hours, and the half-life 9.2 versus 10.4 hours (Table 1). In contrast, the concentration of metabolite 13-*cis*-4-oxo-retinoic acid showed a tendency towards accumulation with time. The mean ratio between the area under the curve (AUC 0-infinity) of 13-*cis*-4-oxo-retinoic acid and 13-*cis* RA rose from 3.4±1 to 5.1±1, and the half-life of the metabolite was 24.5 hours (range 16.5-49.5). Information regarding the pharmacokinetics of 13-*cis* RA during chronic administration was derived from patients who underwent long-term treatment (10 to 360 mg for at least 2 months) for various dermatological diseases. Maximum drug concentration was reached 1 to 4 hours after administration; the elimination half-life ranged from 10 to 23 hours for 13-*cis* RA and from 20 to 49 hours for 13-*cis*-4-oxo-RA; the mean AUC ratio between the two substances was 3.1±1 (1.7-5.4).

Overall, the available data suggest that the plasma levels of 13-*cis* RA were relatively stable after multiple doses, and that the long-term pharmacokinetic profile can be predicted from single-dose data.

Effects on Plasma Retinol

Although recent animal data have demonstrated that oral administration of many retinoids, including 13-*cis* RA, causes a significant and dose-proportional reduction of plasma retinol levels [39], the clinical data on 13-*cis* RA are not conclusive. Some authors reported no effect on plasma retinol levels after relatively high oral doses, ranging from 3mg/kg daily to 5mg/kg daily [9]. Others reported plasma retinol concentrations below the expected normal range in healthy individuals after 1 to 28 days of treatment [37]. However, the baseline levels were not evaluated in these patients, and lower plasma retinol concentrations may well be attributable to the advanced neoplastic status rather than 13-*cis* RA administration.

Fenretinide (4-HPR)

The pharmacokinetics of N-(4-hydroxyphenyl) retinamide (4-HPR) have been studied in healthy volunteers [40,41] and in cancer patients [3,42,43]. After oral administration, maximum blood concentrations of 4-HPR were reached between 3-4 hours, whereas the maximum concentrations of its main metabolite, N-(4-methoxyphenyl)retinamide (4-MPR) occurred between 8-12 hours. The bioavailability of 4-HPR, like that of other retinoids, has been shown to be enhanced by administration with food, and to be influenced by the composition of the meals [44].

Pharmacokinetics after Single and Multiple doses

Following single oral doses of 25, 75, 150, 300, 500 and 600 mg in healthy subjects, a linear relationship between dose and C_{max} and between dose and AUC was found for both 4-HPR and 4-MPR [40,41]. In these subjects the mean elimination half-life of 4-HPR was 16-20 hours and the half-life of 4-MPR 22 hours. Similar values were found in cancer patients treated with a single oral dose of 300 mg [42]: the half-lives of 4-HPR and 4-MPR were 13.7 and 23.0 hours, respectively.

After multiple daily doses of 150 and 300 mg for 28 days (data on file, R.W. Johnson Pharmaceutical Research Institute), no significant differences in the pharmacokinetics of 4-HPR were found between the first and last doses, with a 4-HPR half-life of 27.2 hours. The metabolite 4-MPR showed evidence of accumulation, since the AUC after multiple dosing was higher than for the single dose. Its half-life was 45.1 hours. No unchanged compound, 4-MPR or conjugates were detected in urine [40,41], which is an indication of biliary excretion.

Monitoring of 4-HPR pharmacokinetics during long-term administration has been performed in breast cancer patients who participated in the phase I study of this drug [43] and who were treated for 5 years as the patient group of an ongoing phase III trial [3]. After 5 months of daily treatment with 100, 200 and 300 mg/day doses, a linear relationship was found between the doses administered and the plasma concentrations of both 4-HPR and 4-MPR (Fig. 6) [43]. Daily administration of a dose of 200 mg for 5 years resulted in 4-HPR plasma concentrations of approximately 1 μmol/l, which remained steady during the whole period (Fig. 7) [3].The concentrations of 4-MPR, similar to

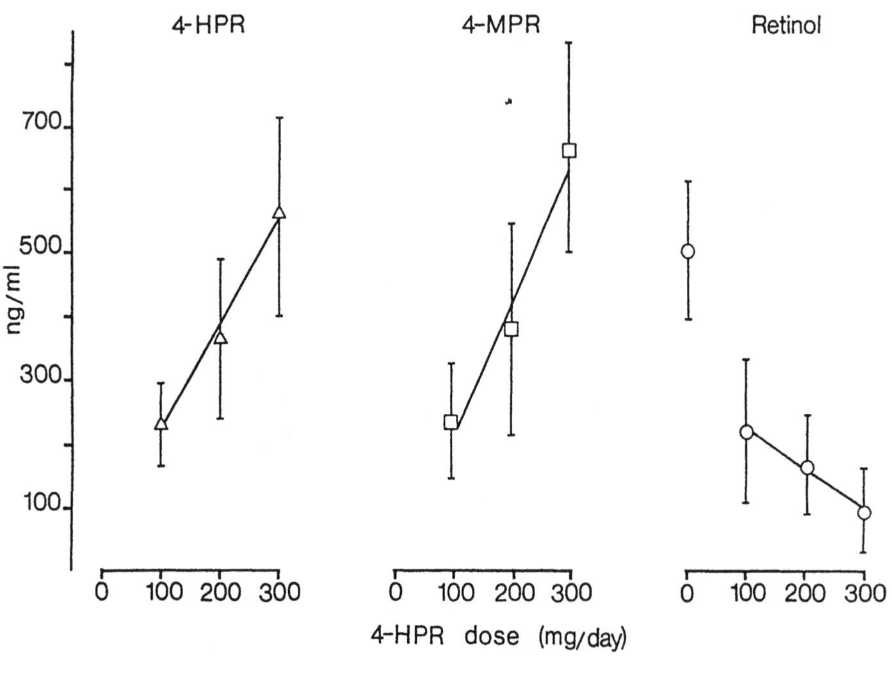

Fig. 6. Relationship between 4-HPR doses (mg/day) and 4-HPR, 4-MPR and retinol plasma levels at 12 hours after 5 months of daily administration. *Points*, mean; *bars*, SD. Reproduced with permission from [43]

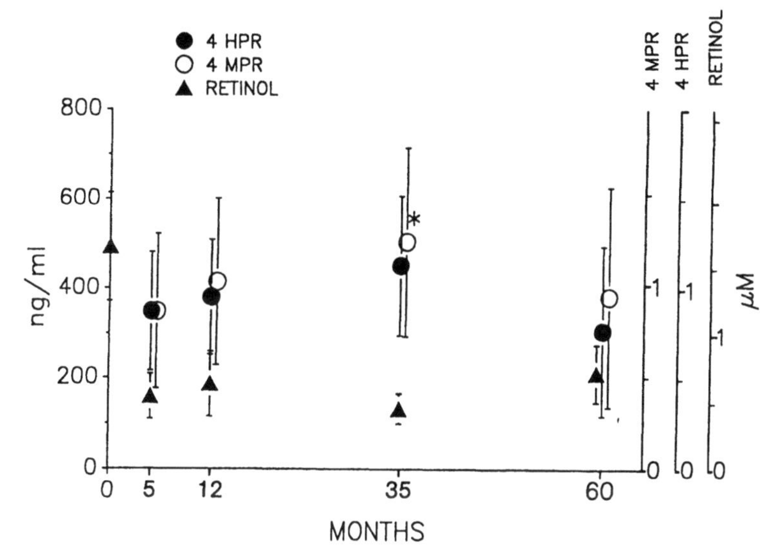

Fig. 7. Mean ± SD plasma concentrations of 4-HPR (●), 4-MPR (○), and retinol (▲) during 5-year chronic treatment. Plasma of 7 patients was collected 14 hours (range, 12-19) after the last drug intake at 5, 12, 35, and 60 months. Baseline retinol concentrations are also reported. *$p < .05$ Dunnet's test vs. 5 months. Reproduced with permission from [3]

those of the parent drug, increased slightly but significantly during the first 35 months and declined thereafter to levels which were not statistically different from those at 5 months. After treatment interruption, in patients treated for 5 years the half-lives of 4-HPR and 4-MPR were 27 and 54 hours, respectively, similar to those found after 28 daily treatments. The findings of constant concentrations and constant half-lives suggest that the pharmacokinetics of this retinoid do not change during-long term treatment, in marked contrast to the situation with all-*trans* retinoid acid. Long-term elimination in patients following completion of 5 years of continuous treatment has also been investigated [3]. At 6 and 12 months after drug discontinuation, the concentrations of 4-HPR were at the limit of detectability (0.01 μmol/l), whereas those of 4-MPR were 5 times higher.

Effects on Plasma Retinol and Retinol Binding Protein

A relevant pharmacological effect of 4-HPR, reported in rats [45] and in humans [42,43,46], is the rapid decrease in the plasma concentrations of both retinol (Fig. 6) and its plasma transport protein RBP [42,43]. The reduction, which is reversible, occurs after a single dose, and is proportional to the dose administered (Fig. 6) [43]. This phenomenon, and its dose dependency, are associated with impaired dark adaptation, a side-effect reported in 4-HPR-treated patients [47-51]. In order to avoid its occurrence, it was decided to incorporate, in the patients of the ongoing prevention trials [52, 53], a 3-day treatment interruption at the end of each month in order to increase plasma retinol concentrations, thus allowing storage of retinol in the retina. During daily treatment with 200 mg 4-HPR, baseline retinol levels were reduced by 71%; after the 3-day drug interruption all patients had recovered clinically, and the mean reduction of retinol levels was 38% [3]. The level of retinol reduction was steady during 5-year continuous treatment (Fig. 7); 1 month after treatment discontinuation the retinol plasma concentrations increased in all patients [3]. Studies performed on the mechanisms responsible for retinol level reduction by 4-HPR have shown that this effect is associated with the high binding affinity of this retinoid to RBP and with its interaction with the RBP-transthyretin (TTR) complex formation [39,54], possibly interfering with secretion of retinol-RBP by the liver or other tissues [55].
A further important biological effect of 4-HPR, which might be related to its chemopreventive activity, is the reduction, recently reported in breast cancer patients [56], of the circulating levels of IGF-I, a potent mitogen for transformed breast epithelial cells.

Concentration in Specific Tissues

Evaluation of 4-HPR concentrations in breast biopsies of some patients [3,57] confirms the ability of this retinoid to accumulate in the breast as previously reported in rodents [58]. The tissue concentrations of 4-HPR were higher (1.4-8.2 times) than those found in plasma. Evidence that this retinoid accumulates not only in the fatty tissue but also in the epithelial cells of the breast is provided by the fact that the concentrations of 4-HPR and 4-MPR in the nipple discharge, which is secreted by the breast gland, were 10 and 30 times higher, respectively, than those found in plasma [3].

Acknowledgement

This work was supported in part by grants FD-R-000764 from the Orphan Products Division, U.S. Food and Drug Administration; by CA-57645 from the U.S. National Cancer Institute; by CA-38567-07 from the U.S. National Cancer Institute.

REFERENCES

1 Muindi J, Frankel S, Huselton C et al: Clinical pharmacology of oral all-trans retinoic acid in patients with acute promyelocytic leukemia. Cancer Res 1992 (52):2138-2142

2 Brazzell RK, Vane FM, Ehmann CW, Colburn WA: Pharmacokinetics of isotretinoin during repetitive dsing to patients. Eur J Clin Pharmacol 1983 (24): 695-702

3 Formelli F, Clerici M, Campa T et al: Five-year administration of fenretinide: pharmacokinetics and effects on plasma retinol concentrations. J Clin Oncol 1993 (11):2036-2042

4 Massarella JW and Vane FM: Etretinate kinetics during chronic dosing in severe psoriasis. Clin Pharmacol Ther 1985 (37):439-446

5 Wiegand UW, Busslinger AA, Chou RC, Jensen BK: The pharmacokinetics of acitretin in humans: an update. In: Livrea MA and Packer L (eds) Retinoids. Progress in Research and Clinical Application. Marcel Dekker Inc, New York 1993 pp 617-628

6 Goodman DS: Vitamin A and retinoids in health and disease. N Engl J Med 1984 (310):1023-1031

7 Blomhoff R, Green MH, Green JB, Berg T, Norum KR: Vitamin A metabolism: new perspectives on absorption, transport and storage. Physiol Rev 1991 (71):951-990

8 Wald NJ, Cuckle HS, Barlow RD et al: The effect of vitamin A supplementation on serum retinol and retinol-binding protein levels. Cancer Lett 1985 (29): 203-213

9 Goodman GE, Alberts DS, Peng YM et al: Pharmacokinetics and phase I trial of retinol and 13-cis-retinoic acid. In: Meyskens FL and Prasad KN (eds) Modulation and Mediation of Cancer by Vitamins. Karger, Basel 1983 pp 311-316

10 Plezia PM, Alberts DS, Peng YM et al: The role of serum and tissue pharmacology studies in the design and interpretation of chemoprevention trials. Preventive Medicine 1989 (18):680-687

11 Infante M, Pastorino U, Chiesa G et al: Laboratory evaluation during high-dose vitamin A administration: a randomised study on lung cancer patients after surgical resection. J Cancer Res Clin Oncol 1991 (117):156-162

12 Korner WF and Vollm J: New aspects of the tolerance of retinol in humans. Int J Vit Nutr Res 1975 (45):363-372

13 Fidge NH, Shiratori T, Ganguly J, Goodman DS: Pathways of absorption of retinal and retinoic acid in the rat. J Lipid Res 1968 (9):103-109

14 Wathne KO, Norum KR, Smeland E, Blomhoff R: Retinol bound to physiological carrier molecules regulates growth and differentiation of myeloid leukemic cells. J Biol Chem 1988 (263):8691-8695

15 Pastorino U, Chiesa G, Infante M et al: Safety of high-dose vitamin A. Randomized trial on lung cancer chemoprevention. Oncology 1991 (48):131-137

16 Huang ME, Ye YC, Chen JR et al: Use of all-trans retinoic acid in the treatment of acute promyelocytic leukemia. Blood 1988 (72):567-572

17 Castaigne S, Chomienne C, Daniel MT et al: All-trans retinoic acid as a differentiation therapy for acute promyelocytic leukemia: I. Clinical results. Blood 1990 (76):1704-1709

18 Warrell RP Jr, Frankel SR, Miller WH Jr et al: Differentiation therapy of acute promyelocytic leukemia with tretinoin (all-trans retinoic acid). N Engl J Med 1991 (324):1385-1393

19 Ohno R, Yoshida H, Naoe T et al: All-trans retinoic acid (ATRA) as a differentiation therapy for refractory acute promyelocytic leukemia (APL). Proc Am Assoc Cancer Res 1992 (33):234

20 White KL, Wiley JS, Frost T et al: All-trans retinoic acid in the treatment of acute promyelocytic leukaemia. Aust NZ J Med 1992 (22):449-454

21 Fenaux P, Le Dely MC, Castaigne S et al: Effect of all-trans retinoic acid in newly diagnosed acute promyelocytic leukemia: results of a multicenter randomized trial. Blood 1993 (82);3241-3249

22 Warrell RP Jr, de Thé H, Wang Z-Y, Degos L: Acute promyelocytic leukemia. N Engl J Med 1993 (329):177-189

23 Frankel SR, Eardley A, Heller G et al: All-trans retinoic acid for acute promyelocytic leukemia: results of the New York study. Ann Intern Med 1994 (120):278-286

24 Fenaux P, Castaigne S, Dombret H et al: All-trans retinoic acid followed by intensive chemotherapy gives a high complete remission rate and may prolong remissions in newly diagnosed acute promyelocytic leukemia: a pilot study on 26 cases. Blood 1992 (80):2176-2181

25 Muindi J, Frankel SR, Miller WH Jr et al: Continuous treatment with all-trans retinoic acid causes a progressive reduction in plasma concentrations: implications for relapse and retinoid "resistance" in patients with acute promyelocytic leukemia. Blood 1992 (79):299-303

26 Delva L, Cornic M, Balitrand N et al: Resistance to all-trans retinoic acid (ATRA) therapy in relapsing acute promyelocytic leukemia: study of in vitro ATRA sensitivity and cellular retinoic acid binding protein levels in leukemic cells. Blood 1993 (82):2175-2181

27 Cornic M, Delva L, Guidez F, Balitrand N, Degos L, Chomienne C: Induction of retinoic acid-binding protein in normal and malignant human myeloid cells by retinoic acid in acute promyelocytic leukemia patients. Cancer Res 1992 (52):3329-3334

28 Lefebvre P, Thomas G, Gourmel B et al: Pharmacokinetics of oral all-trans retinoic acid in patients with acute promyelocytic leukemia. Leukemia 1991 (5):1054-1058

29 Rigas JR, Francis PA, Muindi JRF et al: Constitutive variability in catabolism of the natural retinoid, all-trans retinoic acid, and its modulation by ketoconazole. JNCI 1993 (85):1921-1926

30 Miller VA, Rigas JR, Muindi JRF et al: Modulation of all-trans retinoic acid pharmacokinetics by liarazole. Cancer Chemother Pharmacol 1994 (in press)

31 Muindi JF and Young CW: Lipid hydroperoxides greatly increase the rate of oxidative catabolism of all-trans retinoic acid by human cell culture microsomes genetically enriched in specified cytochrome P-450 isoforms. Cancer Res 1993 (53):1226-1229

32 Fiorella PD and Napoli JL: Expression of cellular

retinoic acid binding protein (CRABP) in *Escherichia coli*: Characterization and evidence that holo-CRABP is a substrate in retinoic acid metabolism. J Biol Chem 1991 (266):16572-16579

33 Boylan JF and Gudas LJ: The level of CRABP-I expression influences the amounts and types of all-trans retinoic acid metabolites in F9 teratocarcinoma stem cells. J Biol Chem 1992 (267):21486

34 Warrell RP Jr: Acquired retinoid resistance in acute promyelocytic leukemia: new mechanisms, strategies, and implications. Blood 1993 (82):1949-1953

35 Robertson KA, Emami B, Collins SJ: Retinoic acid-resistant HL-60R cells harbor a point mutation in the retinoic acid receptor ligand-binding domain that confers dominant negative activity. Blood 1992 (80):1885-1889

36 Dermine S, Grignani F, Clerici M et al: Occurrence of resistance to retinoic acid in the acute promyelocytic cell line NB306 is associated with altered expression of the PML/RAR-a protein. Blood 1994 (in press)

37 Kerr IG, Lippman ME, Jenkins J, Myers C: Pharmacology of 13-cis-retinoic acid in humans. Cancer Res 1982 (42):2069-2073

38 Khoo KC, Reik FD, Colburn WA: Pharmacokinetic profile of isotretinoin following a single oral dose to normal man. J Clin Pharmacol 1982 (22):395-402

39 Berni R, Clerici M, Malpeli G, Cleris L, Formelli F: Retinoids: in vitro interaction with retinol-binding protein and influence on plasma retinol. FASEB J 1993 (7):1179-1184

40 Desiraju RK, Scott V, Nayak RK, Minn FL: Pharmacokinetics of fenretinide in healthy volunteers. Clin Pharmacol Ther 1985 (37/2):190

41 Johnson & Johnson: Fenretinide. Drugs of the Future 1987 (12/3):305-306

42 Peng YM, Dalton WS, Alberts DS et al: Pharmacokinetics of N-4-hydroxyphenyl-retinamide and the effect of its oral administration on plasma retinol concentrations in cancer patients. Int J Cancer 1989 (43):22-26 Erratum: Int J Cancer 1989 (44):567

43 Formelli F, Carsana R, Costa A et al: Plasma retinol level reduction by the synthetic retinoid fenretinide: a one year follow-up study of breast cancer patients. Cancer Res 1989 (49):6149-6152

44 Doose DR, Minn FL, Stellar S, Nayak RK: Effects of meals and meal composition on the bioavailability of fenretinide. J Clin Pharmacol 1992 (32):1089-1095

45 Formelli F, Carsana R, Costa A: N-(4hydroxyphenyl)retinamide (4-HPR) lowers plasma retinol levels in rats. Med Sci Res 1987 (15):843-844

46 Dimitrov NV, Meyer CJ, Perloff M et al: Alteration of retinol-binding-protein concentrations by the synthetic retinoid fenretinide in healthy human subjects. Am J Clin Nutr 1990 (51):1082-1087

47 Kaiser-Kupfer MI, Peck GL, Caruso RC: Abnormal retinal function associated with fenretinide, a synthetic retinoid. Arch Ophtalmol 1986 (104):69-70

48 Costa A, Malone W, Perloff M et al: Tolerability of the synthetic retinoid fenretinide (HPR). Eur J Cancer Clin Oncol 1989 (25):805-808

49 Kingstone TP, Lowe NJ, Winston J, Heckenlively J: Visual and cutaneous toxicity which occurs during n-(4hydroxyphenyl)retinamide therapy for psoriasis. Clin Exper Dermatol 1986 (11):624-627

50 Modiano RM, Dalton WS, Lippman SM et al: Phase II study of fenretinide (N-[4 hydroxyphenyl]retinamide) in advanced breast cancer and melanoma. Inv New Drugs 1990 (8):317-319

51 Decensi A, Torrisi R, Polizzi A et al: Effect of the synthetic retinoid fenretinide on dark adaptation and the ocular surface. JNCI 1994 (86):105-110

52 Veronesi U, De Palo G, Costa A et al: Chemoprevention of breast cancer with retinoids. JNCI Monogr 1992 (12):93-97

53 Chiesa F, Tradati N, Marazza M et al: Prevention of local relapses and new localisations of oral leukoplakias with the synthetic retinoid fenretinide (4-HPR). Preliminary results. Oral Oncol, Eur J Cancer 1992 (28B):97-102

54 Berni R and Formelli F: In vitro interaction of fenretinide with plasma retinol-binding protein and its functional consequences. FEBS 1992 (308):43-45

55 Smith JH, Carpenter Lawless D, Green MH, Moon RC: Secretion of vitamin A and retinol-binding protein into plasma is depressed in rats by N-(4-hydroxyphenyl)retinamide (Fenretinide). J Nutr 1992 (122):1999-2009

56 Torrisi R, Pensa F, Orengo MA, Catsafados E et al: The synthetic retinoid fenretinide lowers plasma insulin-like growth factor I levels in breast cancer patients. Cancer Res 1993 (53):4769-4771

57 Mehta RG, Moon RC, Hawthorne M, Formelli F, Costa A: Distribution of fenretinide in the mammary gland of breast cancer patients. Eur J Cancer 1991 (27):138-141

58 Moon RC, Thompson HJ, Becci PJ et al: N-(4 hydroxyphenyl)retinamide, a new retinoid for prevention of breast cancer. Cancer Res 1979 (39) :1339-1346

Clinical Toxicology of the Retinoids

Raymond P. Warrell, Jr [1], Ugo Pastorino [2] and Andrea Decensi [3]

1 Department of Medicine, Memorial Sloan-Kettering Cancer Center, 1275 York Avenue, New York, NY 10021, U.S.A.
2 Department of Thoracic Surgery, Istituto Nazionale Tumori, Via Venezian 1, 20133 Milan, Italy
3 Department of Medical Oncology II, Istituto Nazionale per la Ricerca sul Cancro, via Benedetto XV 10, 16132 Genoa, Italy

As a class, the retinoids have many side-effects in common. A list of the most frequently observed reactions in relation to the organ systems affected is given in Table 1. Compared to most other drugs used for cancer chemotherapy, these reactions are relatively mild; however, serious and occasionally fatal reactions have occurred, particularly in patients with acute promyelocytic leukaemia (APL).

General Toxicities

Headache beginning several hours after drug ingestion is the most common side-effect of all-*trans* retinoic acid [1-3], but this effect is less prominent with other retinoids in clinical use. Mild analgesics such as acetaminophen or codeine generally suffice for control of this problem, and the patient usually develops a tolerance to the effect within the first 7 to 10 days of treatment. Intracranial hypertension (pseudotumour cerebri), manifested by papilloedema, severe headache, retinal haemorrhages and concentric visual loss, is a known consequence of vitamin A toxicity. This reaction has been documented in a number of patients treated with all-*trans* retinoic acid who required serial lumbar punctures and high-dose corticosteroids for management. For unclear reasons, children are considerably more sensitive than adults to the CNS effects of all-*trans* retinoic acid, and this effect is dose limiting in children [3].

Dry skin, itching, flaking, nasal stuffiness, xerostomia and cheilitis are frequently observed with the use of both all-*trans* and 13-*cis* retinoic

Table 1. Adverse effects of the retinoids

Skin/mucous membranes	
	Skin dryness, itching, peeling
	Genital excoriations
	Angular cheilitis, lip cracking
Central nervous system	
	Headache
	Intracranial hypertension ("pseudotumour cerebri")
Metabolic	
	Hypertriglyceridaemia
	Hypercholesterolaemia
	Hypercalcaemia
	Tumour lysis syndrome**
Haematological*	
	Marked leukocytosis
	Thrombosis
Gastrointestinal	
	Hepatic toxicity (increased SGOT, alkaline phosphatase, bilirubin)
	Pancreatitis
Cardiovascular*	
	Congestive heart failure
	Fluid overload
	Lower extremity oedema
	Episodic hypotension
	Weight gain
	Pericardial effusion
Pulmonary*	
	Respiratory distress
	Pleural effusion
	Radiographic infiltrates

* Occurs in patients with acute myelocytic leukaemias only

** A rare occurrence in patients with acute promyelocytic leukaemia acid. These reactions have been managed with topical lubricants and moisturising agents; however, some patients (particularly those receiving 13-*cis* RA) may require a decrease in the drug dose due to these effects. Genital ulcerations, especially scrotal excoriations, have been observed with all-*trans* RA [1,4].

Bone pain occurs in 10-20% of APL patients receiving all-*trans* RA [1,4]. This effect tends to appear early during remission induction and usually subsides even when therapy is continued. Occasionally the pain can be quite severe and narcotics may be required for relief. Bone pain is a less prominent problem for patients on 13-*cis* retinoic acid; however, long-term treatment with 13-*cis* RA has been associated with formation of hyperostosis (bone spurs), particularly on the vertebral bodies and in the calcaneus [5,6]. Hypercalcaemia has also been reported occasionally [7,8].

Hypertriglyceridaemia has been observed with most retinoids, but hypercholesterolaemia is less striking [1,9]. Cardiovascular consequences specifically related to hyperlipidaemia have not yet been described; however, such complications may assume increasing importance as these agents are used for more extended periods or for cancer chemoprevention. Pancreatitis has been described in association with hypertriglyceridaemia [10]. Hypolipidaemic agents have not been systematically investigated for their utility in ameliorating these effects.

Hepatic toxicity is a well-known side-effect of all retinoids. Generally this effect is manifested by a transient increase in serum transaminases, alkaline phosphatase, or bilirubin during the first weeks of therapy. Although these effects may persist for several weeks after the drugs have been discontinued, the changes are usually readily reversible on cessation of therapy.

The use of all-*trans* retinoic acid in APL has been associated with thrombosis [11]; however, it is unclear whether this effect is due to the coagulopathy associated with this form of leukaemia or to the drug itself. An increased incidence of thrombosis has not been reported in other diseases nor with other retinoids. In rare cases a syndrome of hyperhistaminaemia associated with extreme basophilia has been observed in patients with acute promyelocytic leukaemia during therapy with all-*trans* RA [12].

As a group the retinoids are exceptionally potent teratogens, an extension of their physiological role in morphogenesis. This potential side-effect has been a particular concern in retinoid treatment of non-malignant dermatological conditions such as acne and psoriasis. However, both APL and breast cancer can occur in a relatively young age group; therefore, a pregnancy test should be performed prior to therapeutic use in women of child-bearing age and adequate contraception should be practiced during therapy. The risk of foetal malformation appears to be highest in the first trimester and quite low in the third trimester [13-15].

The clinical experience with 9-cis retinoic acid and 3-methyl TTNEB is too limited to draw any conclusions regarding the side-effects specifically associated with these compounds.

Leukocytosis and the "Retinoic Acid Syndrome" in APL

Two important problems have been noted in the treatment of patients with acute promyelocytic leukaemia. The first is leukocytosis (defined as an increase in peripheral leukocytes >20,000 cells/mm^3), which may occur in almost one half of APL patients treated with all-*trans* retinoic acid [16,17]. Although the development of leukocytosis was originally equated with an unfavourable outcome [18], additional experience has indicated that an increase in the peripheral blood leukocyte count is usually the first clinical indication of a biological response. These early cells comprise a spectrum of myeloid cells including myeloblasts, promyelocytes, "intermediate cells" and granulocytes, most of which are derived from the leukaemic clone and eventually eliminated [1]. In most patients, the coagulopathy of APL disappears early and does not reappear despite the increased leukocyte count. Accordingly, additional cytotoxic therapy specifically directed toward lowering the leukocyte count is not indicated in most patients. Such treatment may in fact be hazardous since even low-dose chemotherapy (hydroxyurea or cytosine arabinoside) has been a triggering event for lethal coagulopathy in some patients [17].

Approximately 20% of patients with APL treated with all-*trans* retinoic acid have experienced the so-called "retinoic acid syndrome", a condition characterised by high fever, respiratory distress, radiographic pulmonary infiltrates, weight gain, and pleural or pericardial effusions [16]. Although originally attributed to pneumonia or congestive heart failure, this reaction is now seen as a characteristic feature of all-*trans* RA treatment in APL and it represents by far the most serious reaction encountered with the use of this agent. Autopsies on patients who died of this problem have shown extensive infiltration of myeloid cells into lungs, skin, kidney, liver and lymph nodes. Although leukocytosis is frequently observed with this syndrome, the onset of the reaction occurs with a relatively normal leukocyte count in up to one-third of cases [4,16]. Early recognition of the syndrome (especially unexplained fever, dyspnoea, or weight gain) is critical, and the appearance of these signs should prompt immediate steroid treatment. Short courses of corticosteroids (dexamethasone 10 mg i.v. every 12 hours for 3 or more days) have been used, and this therapy has reversed progression of the syndrome in most patients [16,17]. The clinician should employ a low threshold for steroid treatment; in a recent series, up to 50% of patients were treated with almost complete protection from the syndrome and no important sequelae other than hyperglycaemia.

The role of chemotherapy during induction therapy of APL with all-*trans* RA remains controversial. In Europe the approach has been to initiate full-dose chemotherapy (anthracycline plus cytosine arabinoside) if the initial leukocyte count is greater than 5,000/mm^3 or if the count exceeds 5,000 cells/mm^3 on day 6, 10,000/mm^3 on day 10, or 15,000/mm^3 on day 15. However, this approach has not reduced early mortality relative to patients treated with chemotherapy alone nor has it eliminated the retinoic acid syndrome as a problem [19]. Moreover, this approach has also greatly increased both costs and morbidity compared to patients treated solely with all-*trans* RA [20]. A high initial leukocyte count (e.g. > 20,000/mm^3) remains a poor prognostic feature irrespective of treatment, although some patients appear to have done well with the combined approach [21]. The majority of APL patients do not require additional chemotherapy during induction. The role of such treatment in preventing morbidity and mortality in those individuals whose leukocyte counts rise to very high levels under all-*trans* RA therapy (> 125,000/mm^3) is not yet defined. Although uncommon, a "tumour lysis syndrome" consisting of accelerated intravascular coagulation, hyperphosphataemia and hyperuricaemia, has been observed when these differentiated "intermediate cells" rapidly decrease in the peripheral blood (without the use of chemotherapy); this effect generally occurs after 10 to 20 days of treatment (R.P. Warrell, Jr, unpublished observations). Both leukocytosis and the "retinoic acid syndrome" have occurred in patients with non-APL acute myelocytic leukaemias but not in patients with solid tumours. It is unclear whether clinical trials using all-*trans* RA plus a haematopoietic colony-stimulating factor will increase this incidence.

Ocular Toxicity of Fenretinide

One of the main reasons oncologists are attracted to 4-HPR is its tolerability in comparison to other retinoids. As shown by a randomised phase I study of different doses of 4-HPR [22], no acute or severe toxicity is observed with this retinoid. The same holds for long-term, daily oral administration of 200 mg 4-HPR, as shown by the evaluation of 53 patients treated for 42 months [23]. Dermatologic and metabolic alterations are relatively uncommon (<5%) and no liver function abnormalities have been observed [24]. Occurrence of diminished dark adaptation, however, is more common. Estimation of this secondary effect by the Goldmann-Weekers dark-adaptometry test, which can very sensitively detect subclinical vitamin A deficiency, has shown that there is a 23% incidence of mild and a 26% incidence of moderate alteration of dark-adaptometry associated with the drug-induced decline of plasma retinol below the threshold levels of 160 and 100 ng/ml, respectively, in women treated with 200 mg 4-HPR daily [25]. However, nearly 50% of these treated patients with altered dark-adaptometry are asymptomatic, thus leaving the true clinical significance of the finding unclear. In addition, the alterations of dark-adaptometry are promptly reversible upon drug interruption.

Plasma 4-MPR, the principal metabolite of 4-HPR which is higher in elderly women with a higher percentage of adipose tissue, is the major determinant of decreased retinol, suggesting a possible biological effect of both age and adipose tissue on the toxicologic profile of this retinoid [26]. This subgroup may warrant more careful ophthalmologic surveillance. Toxicity of the ocular surface, frequently observed with administration of natural and synthetic retinoids [27], is negligible in 4-HPR-treated patients [25].

Acknowledgement

This work was supported in part by grants FD-R-000764 from the Orphan Products Division, U.S. Food and Drug Administration; by CA-57645 from the U.S. National Cancer Institute.

REFERENCES

1 Warrell RP Jr, de Thé H, Wang Z-Y, Degos L: Acute promyelocytic leukemia. N Engl J Med 1993 (329): 177-189

2 Lee JS, Newman RA, Lippman SM et al: Phase I evaluation of all-trans retinoic acid in adults with solid tumors. J Clin Oncol 1993 (11):959

3 Smith MA, Adamson PC, Balis FM et al: Phase I and pharmacokinetic evaluation of all-trans retinoic acid in pediatric patients with cancer. J Clin Oncol 1992 (10):1666-1673

4 Frankel SR, Eardley A, Heller G, Berman E, Warrell RP Jr: All-trans retinoic acid for acute promyelocytic leukemia: results of the New York study. Ann Intern Med 1994 (120):278-286

5 DiGiovanna J, Helfgott R, Gerber L et al: Extraspinal tendon and ligament calcification associated with long-term therapy with etretinate. N Engl J Med 1986 (315):1177-1182

6 Kilcoyne R: Effects of retinoids on bone. J Am Acad Dermatol 1988 (19):212-216

7 Akiyama H, Nakamura N, Nagasaka S, Sakamaki H, Onozawa Y: Hypercalcaemia due to all-trans retinoic acid. Lancet 1992 (339):308-309

8 Niesvizky R, Siegel D, Straus D et al: Hypercalcemia and increased serum interleukin-6 (IL-6) levels induced by all-trans retinoic acid (ATRA) in patients with multiple myeloma. Proc Am Soc Clin Oncol 1993 (12):407

9 Warrell RP Jr, Frankel SR, Miller WH Jr et al: Differentiation therapy of acute promyelocytic leukemia with tretinoin (all-trans retinoic acid). N Engl J Med 1991 (324):1385-1393

10 Izumi T, Hatake K, Miura Y: Acute promyelocytic leukemia (letter). New Engl J Med 1994 (330):141

11 Runde V, Aul C, Sudhoft T, Heyll A, Schneider W: Retinoic acid in the treatment of acute promyelocytic leukemia: Inefficacy of the 13-cis isomer and induction of complete remission by the all-trans isomer complicated by thromboembolic events. Ann Hematol 1992 (64):270-272

12 Koike T, Tatewaki W, Aoki A et al: Severe symptoms of hyperhistaminemia after the treatment of acute promyelocytic leukemia with tretinoin (all-trans retinoic acid). New Engl J Med 1992 (327): 385-387

13 Lammer EJ, Chen DT, Hoar RM et al: Retinoic acid fetopathy. N Engl J Med 1985 (313):837-841

14 Dai WS, LaBraico JM, Stern RS: Epidemiology of isotretinoin exposure during pregnancy. J Am Acad Dermatol 1992 (26):599-560

15 Jick SS, Terris BZ, Jick H: First trimester topical tretinoin and congenital disorders. Lancet 1993 (341):1181-1182

16 Frankel SR, Eardley A, Lauwers G, Weiss M, Warrell RP Jr: The "retinoic acid syndrome" in acute promyelocytic leukemia. Ann Intern Med 1992 (117):292-296

17 Vadhat L, Eardley A, Heller G, Warrell RP Jr: Leukocytosis, the retinoic acid syndrome, and early mortality in acute promyelocytic leukema: when is chemotherapy needed during remission induction with all-trans retinoic acid. Blood 1993 (82 suppl):192A

18 Castaigne S, Chomienne C, Fenaux P, Daniel MT, Degos L: Hyperleukocytosis during all-trans retinoic acid for acute promyelocytic leukemia. Blood 1990 (76 suppl):260a

19 Fenaux P, Le Dely MC, Castaigne S et al: Effect of all-trans retinoic acid in newly diagnosed acute promyelocytic leukemia: results of a multicenter randomized trial. Blood 1993 (82):3241-3249

20 Eardley AM, Heller G, Warrell RP Jr: Morbidity and costs of all-trans retinoic acid compared to standard chemotherapy for remission induction in acute promyelocytic leukemia. Leukemia 1994 (8):934-939

21 Dombret H, Sutton L, Duarte M, Daniel MT, Leblond V, Castaigne S et al: Combined therapy with all-trans retinoic acid and high-dose chemotherapy in patients with hyperleukocytic acute promyelocytic leukemia and severe visceral hemorrhage. Leukemia 1992 (6):1237-1242

22 Costa A, Malone W, Perloff M et al: Tolerability of the synthetic retinoid fenretinide (HPR). Eur J Cancer Clin Oncol 1989 (25):805-808

23 Rotmensz N, De Palo G, Formelli F et al: Long term tolerability of fenretinide (4-HPR) in breast cancer patients. Eur J Cancer 1991 (2):1127-1131

24 Pizzichetta M, Rossi R, Costa A et al: Lipoproteins in fenretinide (4-HPR) treated patients. Diab Nutr Metab 1992 (5):71-72

25 Decensi A, Torrisi R, Polizzi A et al: Effect of the synthetic retinoid fenretinide on dark-adaptation and the ocular surface. JNCI 1994 (86):105-110

26 Torrisi R, Parodi S, Fontana V et al: Factors affecting plasma retinol decline during long-term administration of the synthetic retinoid Fenretinide in breast cancer patients. Cancer Epidemiol Biomarkers & Prev 1994 (3):507-510

27 Gross EG and Helfgott MA: Retinoids and the eye. Dermatol Clin 1992 (10):521-531

Clinical and Molecular Advances in Acute Promyelocytic Leukaemia

Hugues de Thé 1, Laurent Degos 1 and Raymond P. Warrell, Jr 2

1 Institut Universitaire d'Hématologie, Hôpital St. Louis, 1, Avenue Claude Vellefaux, 75010 Paris, France
2 Department of Medicine, Memorial Sloan-Kettering Cancer Center, 1275 York Avenue, New York, NY 10021, U.S.A.

Acute promyelocytic leukaemia (APL) comprises approximately 10% of the acute myeloblastic leukaemias in adults [1,2]. The disease was first recognised as a distinctive clinical entity in the 1950s [3] and it typically presents with a severe bleeding diathesis that is exacerbated by chemotherapy [4-7]. This feature has led to a relatively high rate of early mortality, ranging from 8% to 47% in recent series [4-9], primarily as a consequence of intracranial haemorrhage [9-11]. In this chapter, we review the latest information regarding the molecular genetics and current methods of therapy of this disease.

Molecular Genetics of Acute Promyelocytic Leukaemia

In leukaemia, chromosomal translocations are thought to contribute to carcinogenesis generally by causing either deregulated expression of an otherwise intact oncogene or fusion of two genes that leads to production of a chimaeric protein with new functional properties. In 1977, APL was shown to be consistently associated with a non-random chromosomal abnormality characterised by balanced and reciprocal translocations between the long arms of chromosomes 15 and 17, namely t(15;17)(q22;q11-21) [12-14]. In 1987, the retinoic acid receptor α (RAR-α) was shown to map to chromosome 17 at position q21 [15]. The breakpoint location and the coincident demonstration of the clinical activity of all-*trans* retinoic acid in APL suggested that RAR-α might be involved in this translocation. This finding prompted an analysis of the involved gene's structure and expression; several groups then showed that RAR-α was rearranged in virtually all patients tested [16-20]. Subsequently, the t(15;17) breakpoint was cloned, which showed that the abnormality on chromosome 15 tightly clustered in a region that contained a previously unknown gene, initially called *myl,* later renamed PML (for promyelocytic leukaemia) [21-32]. A chimaeric mRNA was transcribed from the translocated chromosome that yielded a PML/RAR-α fusion protein. Thus, in APL as in certain other diseases, a chromosomal translocation generates a disease-specific fusion protein that is presumably involved in carcinogenesis [33].

RAR-α (and possibly PML) are transcription factors, and this finding strongly suggests that the fusion protein transforms cells through deregulation of transcriptional control (see below) [34]. However, the paradoxical observation of an altered retinoic acid receptor inducing a disease responsive to retinoic acid raises a number of questions as to the potential molecular mechanism(s) that may be involved. The use of all-*trans* retinoic acid as a treatment for APL is the prime example to date of a therapy targeted at a defined genetic lesion in a human cancer. Moreover, this therapeutic approach is based on the induction of cytodifferentiation and as such it represents the first consistently successful example of differentiation therapy. For both these reasons, APL has become a key model system in cancer biology [35].

The amino-acid sequence of PML points to important structural motifs: a zinc finger domain (which could be a DNA- or protein-binding motif common to a large group of proteins [36]), and a leucine zipper dimerisation motif. Since both of these domains are commonly found in transcription factors, it has been proposed that PML itself belongs to this family of nuclear proteins. The presence of these two regions also defines a subfamily of 7 members that include oncogenes, transcription factors and a component of the ribonucleoprotein complex found as an autoantigen in lupus erythematosus [37]. Interestingly, immunofluorescence studies have shown that several members of this family have a speckled nuclear pattern of expression as they are bound to discrete nuclear domains. The localisation of the PML protein is similarly nuclear with a speckled distribution that results from the binding of the protein to a so-called "nuclear body" [38-40]. Nuclear bodies can be detected by electron microscopy and they react with certain autoantibodies (principally those arising in primary biliary cirrhosis). The function of nuclear bodies is unknown, but they are abundant in hormone or lectin-activated cells. Within the PML gene family, two other members are, like PML, also deleted and fused to other genes during oncogenic activation, a finding that further suggests these structural alterations are oncogenic.

The 15;17 translocation results in the synthesis of 2 reciprocal fusion transcripts, PML/RAR-α (found in all cases studied to date) and RAR-α/PML (found in about two-thirds of cases). The PML/RAR-α fusion protein contains all functional domains of PML and RAR-α (i.e. the N-terminal portion of PML, including the zinc finger and leucine zipper regions, is fused to the DNA-binding and hormone-binding domains of RAR-α) (Fig. 1). While the RAR-α breakpoints on chromosome 17 always occur in intron 2 (including deletion of the N-terminal end of RAR-α known as the A region), the breakpoints on chromosome 15 cluster in two different introns and one exon of PML, leading to distinct fusion proteins (Fig. 1). Differences in the PML breakpoint location have not correlated with patient survival, cellular morphology, cell surface antigen expression, sex, or age.

In very rare cases that by morphology appear to have been typical of APL, RAR-α was recently shown to be fused to a zinc finger gene, known as PLZF, as a consequence of an 11;17 chromsomal translocation [41]. (Interestingly, these cases have not been clinically responsive to all-*trans* retinoic acid.) These variant t(11;17) translocations have had the same N-terminal deletion of RAR-α as PML/RAR-α. This region contains an RA-independent transactivation domain that is involved in gene- and tissue-specific activation [42]. The finding that similar fusions of RAR-α occur with two different genes in the same disease strongly suggests that RAR-α alterations themselves are critically involved in the leukaemogenic process.

The detailed structure of the proteins generated from the translocated alleles is quite complex [43]. The PML/RAR-α fusion product can undergo alternative splicing, and PML proteins with C-terminal deletions can be produced. Although the mRNA of the PML/RAR-α fusion is far less abundant in APL cells than that of normal RAR-α, the fusion protein is found in large excess relative to the normal receptor protein encoded by the intact chromosome 17. This excess is likely due to a block in translation of RAR-α mRNA which contains a very long 5'-untranslated sequence. These observations have suggested that the aberrant PML/RAR-α may exert a "dominant" effect over the normal RAR-α gene product (Fig. 1).

The transforming potential of the fusion gene products has not been directly established. Therefore, most investigators have focused upon evaluating other properties of the fusion proteins such as effects on transcription, DNA binding, differentiation, intranuclear traffic, and so forth. In co-transfection assays using RA-sensitive reporter genes, PML/RAR-α has not behaved as a normal retinoic acid receptor, although the type of alteration (repression or overactivation) has varied depending upon the experimental system [27-30]. At the molecular level, several mechanisms could account for this effect of PML/RAR-α. Unlike RAR-α (which requires retinoid "X" receptors [RXRs] as a cofactor), PML/RAR-α can homodimerize via the PML leucine zipper and bind RA-response elements or related DNA sequences [44]. Thus, PML/RAR-α has an altered DNA-binding spectrum and consequently could activate or repress RA-target genes (or other sets of genes). PML/RAR-α also appears to heterodimerize with RXRs. The abundance of PML/RAR-α and its altered localisation (see below) could lead to the sequestration of RXRs away from their normal partners (RARs, thyroid hormone receptors, and vitamin D_3 receptors) and block the function of these normal receptors. Indeed, in stable or transient expression systems, PML/RAR-α was shown to block the

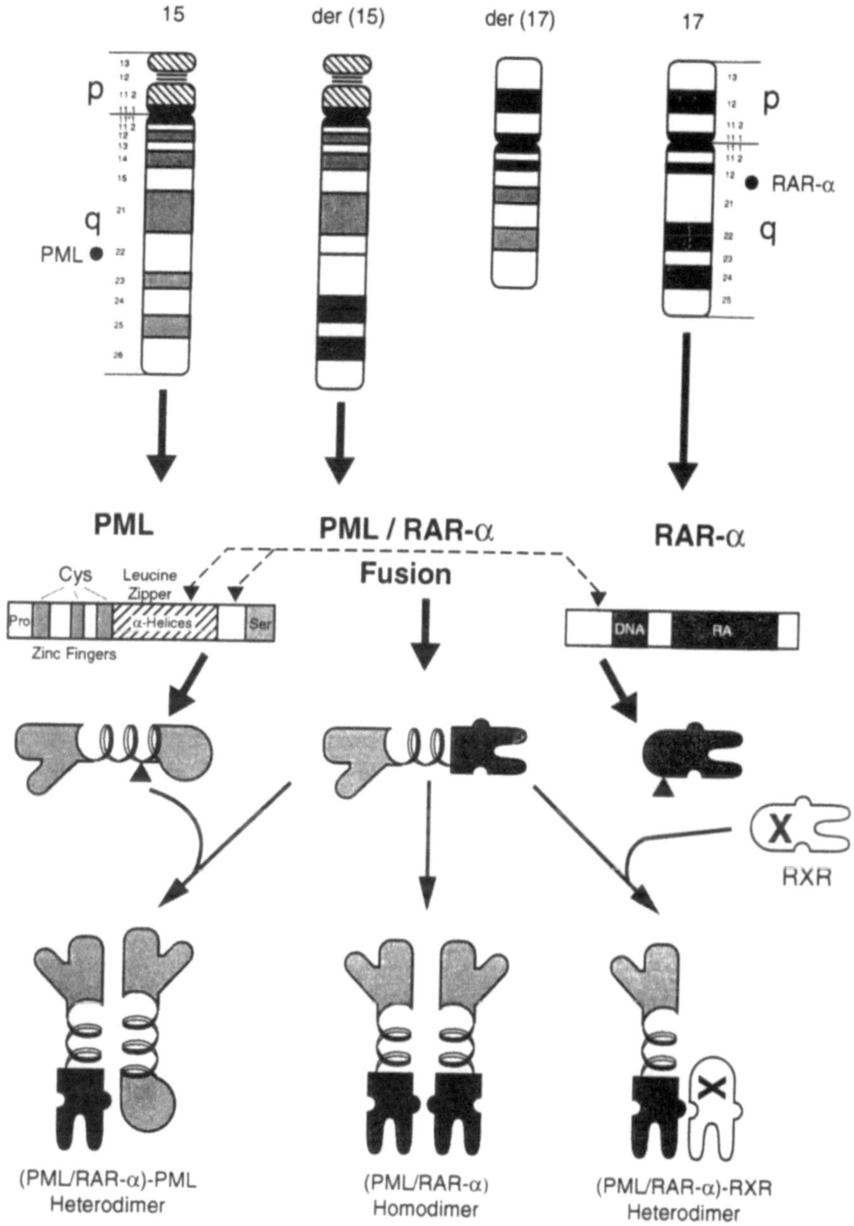

Fig. 1. Diagram depicting sites of the reciprocal translocations between the long (q) arms of chromosomes 15 and 17 in acute promyelocytic leukaemia (outer two chromosomes), leading to breakage and fusion of genes encoding RAR-α and PML, shown in the inner pair of derived (der) chromosomes. In addition to mRNA for normal ("wild-type") RAR-α and PML, the PML/RAR-α fusion mRNA has been transcribed in all cases tested to date, whereas RAR-α/PML has been found in approximately two-thirds of patients. A diagram of the protein sequences in the middle of the figure shows the most common breakpoints (dark triangles) involved in the APL translocations. At the bottom, possible mechanisms are depicted whereby the PML/RAR-α fusion could lead to leukaemogenesis, including heterodimerisation with (and inactivation of) wild-type PML, inactivation of RXR, or homodimerisation of the fusion proteins and subsequent binding to PML or RAR-α target genes. Reprinted with permission from [117]

response to vitamin D_3 (a pathway that is also involved in myeloid differentiation) [44,45]. Whether through sequestration of RXRs, modified DNA-binding specificities, or transactivating properties, PML/RAR-α leads to a global alteration in transcriptional control that may be implicated in leukaemogenesis.

Can these observations account for the proposed leukaemogenic role of the t(15,17) in APL? The differentiating effect of all-*trans* retinoic acid on HL60 cells, as well as work on avian haematopoiesis, suggest that retinoic acid could be involved in normal myeloid differentiation [46-49]. Moreover, RAR-α transdominant mutants impair the differentiation of HL60 cells, certain varieties of immortalised precursor cells, and normal mouse progenitor cells [50-52]. This differentiation block occurs at the promyelocyte stage and is, in part, reversible by retinoic acid. Finally, an avian retroviral oncogene, *v-erbA*, (which is itself an altered thyroid hormone receptor) causes erythroleukaemia in chickens in part by impairing the function of RARs (as shown by transforming *v-erbA* mutants that selectively impair RAR function [53]). These experiments strongly suggest that retinoic acid and RAR-α are implicated in promyelocytic maturation. Thus, the

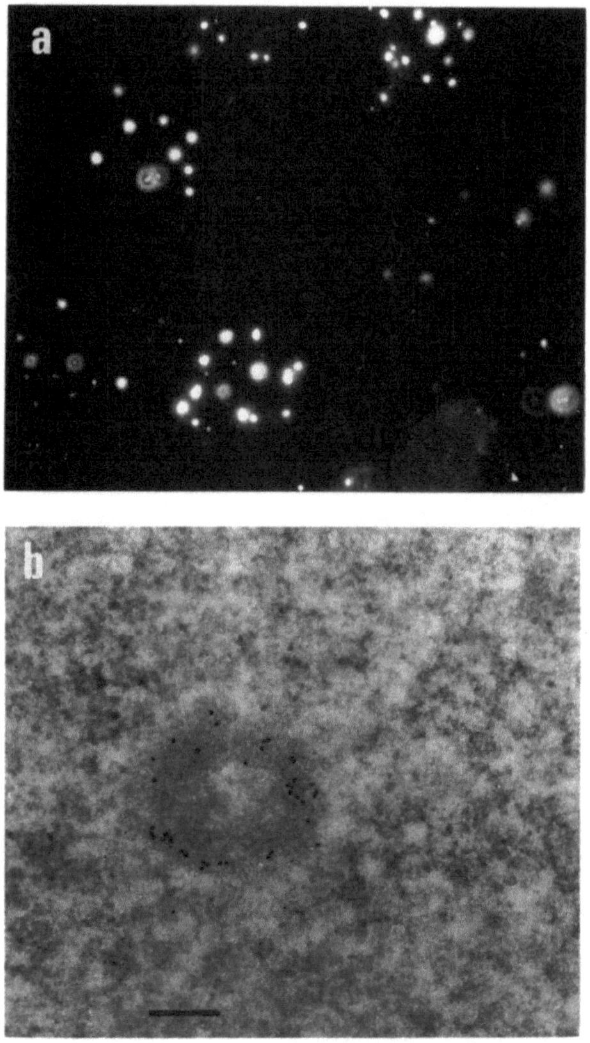

Fig. 2. Specific localisation of PML on a nuclear body. A) Immunofluorescence pattern of PML in fibroblast cells. B) Electron microscopic view of a nuclear body specifically immunolabelled with PML antibodies. Reprinted with permission from [39]

functionally impaired hybrid receptor may contribute to leukaemogenesis by antagonising differentiation. Indeed, several groups have shown that expression of the PML/RAR-α gene in established myeloid cells (U937 or HL60) impairs or blocks myeloid differentiation induced by RA, TGF-ß, or vitamin D_3 [45,54].

An alternative (or complementary) approach comes from the study of the intranuclear localisation of PML and PML/RAR-α [38-40]. Analysis of the localisation of these two gene products in transfected cells had shown that they were located in different cellular compartments (Figs. 2 and 3) [30,38]. While PML was located in nuclear speckles (later identified as nuclear bodies) [55,60], PML/RAR-α was located either in the cytoplasm or in smaller and more numerous nuclear regions of unknown structure. These studies were extended to APL blasts (Fig. 3). PML/RAR-α and PML proteins (presumably as a heterodimer) are located partly in the cytoplasm and partly in the nucleus in microspeckles that are distinct from nuclear bodies. Importantly, other antigens associated with nuclear bodies (such as Sp100) [61] are also scattered from their normal speckled localisation. This finding implies that a large protein complex has an altered nuclear localisation as the result of PML/RAR-α expression. While these experiments imply that the function of these nuclear bodies is most likely impaired, their relevance to leukaemogenesis is as yet unclear due to lack of knowledge regarding the normal role of these structures. The treatment of APL cells with retinoic acid leads to the reaggregation of these antigens onto the nuclear body. The exact mechanism involved (e.g. disruption of PML/RAR-α-PML heterodimers, rerouting of PML/RAR-α) is unclear.

In Figure 4, we propose a model of the traffic of nuclear body antigens in APL. Fusion of a nuclear receptor hormone-binding domain to a transcription factor results in a hormone-dependent function [62]. It was previously proposed that fusion of PML to RAR-α might render PML function RA dependent [27,63]. If indeed PML is a key regulatory gene for promyelocytic differentiation or growth control, impairment and RA dependence of PML function might be relevant to transformation.

The spectacular and highly specific effect of retinoic acid in APL remains relatively poorly understood at the molecular level [64,65]. Several of the above-mentioned abnormalities induced by PML/RAR-α are reversible by retinoic acid. However, the lack of a testable *in vivo* transformation model precludes elucidation of the exact molecular mechanism of leukaemogenesis and the basis of the response to all-*trans* retinoic acid *in vivo*. The observation that cell lines that both carry (NB4) and do not carry (HL60) a chimaeric receptor, respond to retinoic acid in a comparable manner is still puzzling. One central question would be to determine whether the differentiation pathways activated

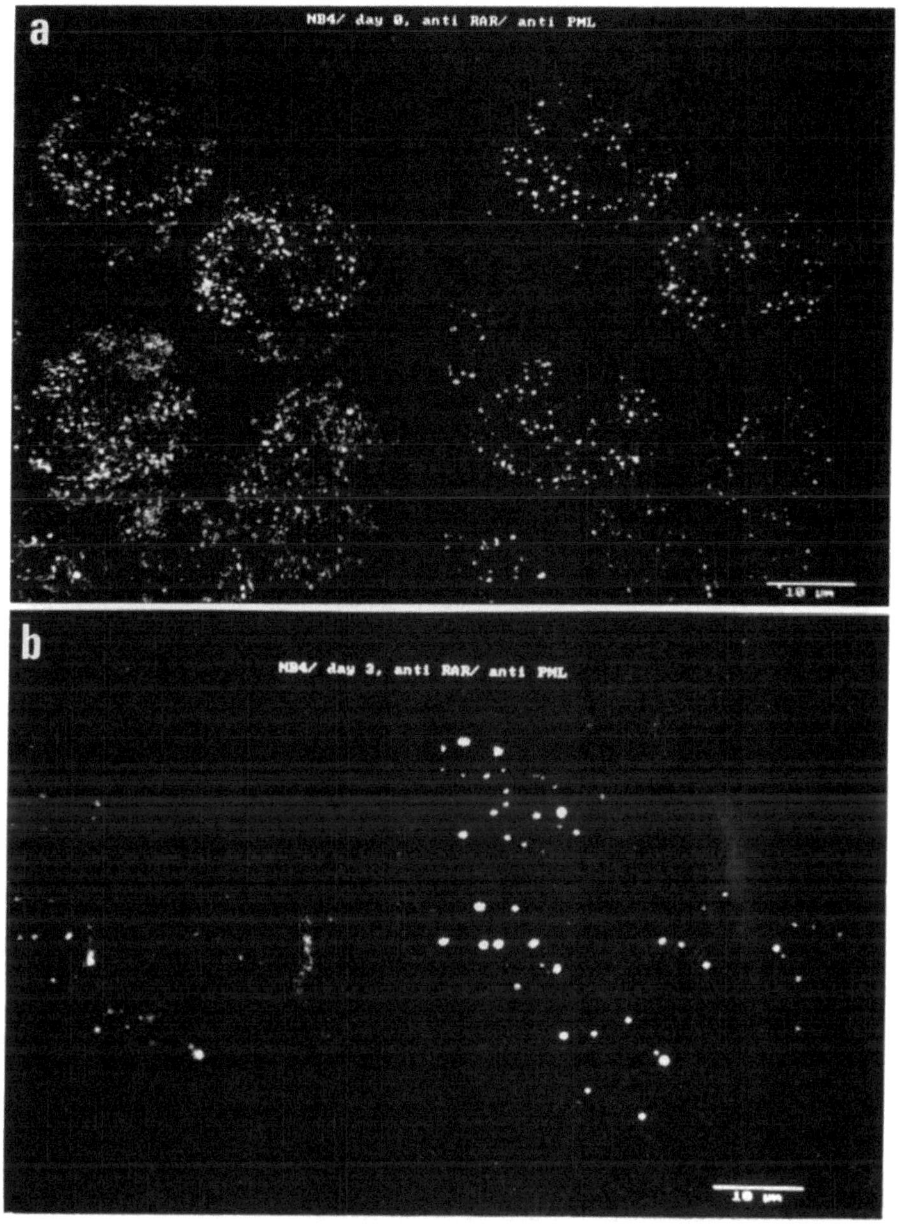

Fig. 3. Expression patterns of PML in APL cells: effect of treatment with all-*trans* retinoic acid. A) Untreated cells. B) NB4 cells following a 72-hour exposure. The left part of the figure represents RAR-α labelling; the right part represents PML labelling revealed by confocal microscopy. Note the modifications in the size of the dots as assessed by PML antibodies and the disappearance of RAR-α labelling after RA therapy. Reprinted with permission from [39]

by administration of retinoic acid in NB4 or HL60 cells are identical, or whether the convergence between the two models is merely incidental.

Clinical Features of Acute Promyelocytic Leukaemia

Certain clinical features have historically been recognised as conferring an adverse prognosis in APL, including leukocytosis, thrombocytopenia, hypofibrinogenaemia, and initial haemorrhage [5,7,66-69]. Several pathological processes are involved in the coagulopathy, including accelerated intravascular coagulation, hyperfibrinolysis, and thrombocytopenia [70]. Individuals may differ in the severity of any single process, and this variability may explain divergent findings among several clinical studies. Clearly, lysis of malignant cells releases procoagulant substances that activate the coagulation cascade, generate thrombin, and cause depletion of fibrinogen, clotting factors, and platelets [71-73]. Hyperfibrinolysis (which may be primary or secondary) may be associated with release of plasminogen activators [74-76] or elastase [77,78], or by the progressive depletion of homeostatic fibrinolytic in-

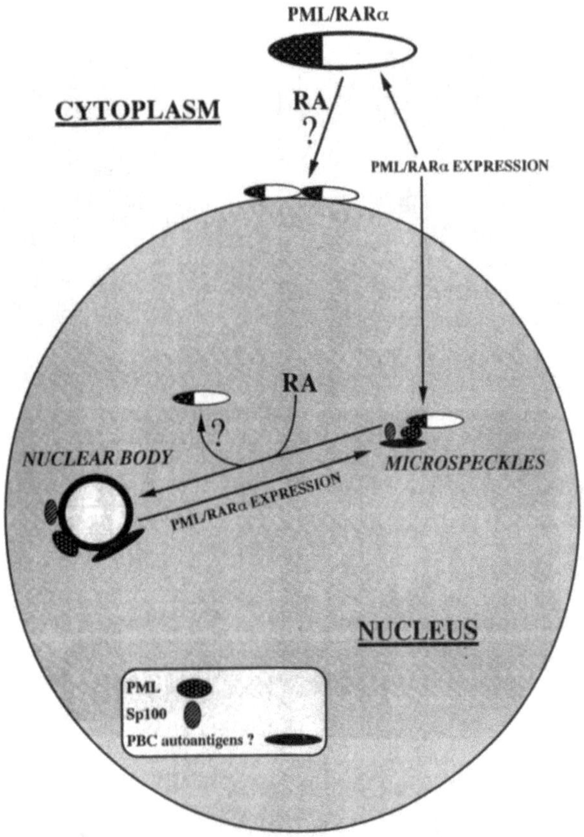

Fig. 4. Proposed scheme of the intranuclear trafficking of nuclear body-associated antigens in APL. Reprinted with permission from [39]

hibitors such as α-$_2$-antiplasmin, plasminogen activator inhibitor, and C1 esterase inhibitor [79-83].

With conventional chemotherapy (e.g. an anthracycline plus cytosine arabinoside), remission can be achieved in 60% to 80% of patients [2,5,6,8,84]. Despite the excess in early mortality, long-term survival in APL is somewhat more favourable relative to other subtypes of acute myeloblastic leukaemia, and survival at 5 years usually ranges from 35% to 45% [5,6,68,85,86]. The benefits of extended maintenance chemotherapy remain controversial [4,6,87].

Clinical Activity of All-*Trans* Retinoic Acid in APL

Early studies by Breitman and colleagues showed that all-*trans* RA and its isomer 13-*cis* RA were equally effective in inducing differentiation of HL60 cells *in vitro* [48]. Notwithstanding several case reports [88-91], considerable clinical experience - much of it unpublished - suggests that positive benefits due to 13-*cis* RA reflect publication bias wherein a small number of positive results are reported and large numbers of negative results are unrecorded. Later studies have indicated that 13-*cis* RA is at least 1 log less effective than all-*trans* RA against fresh human leukaemic cells in culture [92], and recently treated patients have shown no important clinical response [93,94].

The first patients with APL were treated with all-*trans* retinoic acid in Shanghai in 1986 [95]. Since that time, a variety of doses have been employed, ranging from 10 to 100 mg/m^2 of body surface area. Over this dosage range, however, no particular dose-effect correlation has emerged with respect to initial therapeutic response, although formal studies to carefully address this issue have not been conducted. Most clinical experience has been obtained with a dose of 45 mg/m^2 administered once per day or in 2 equally divided doses [93,95-101].

Induction of Remission

As of early 1994, approximately 2,000 patients with a clinical diagnosis of acute promyelocytic leukaemia had been treated world-wide with all-*trans* RA. Table 1 summarises the clinical activity of the drug from results reported in 565 of these cases. Combining data from the Chinese, French, New York, and Nagoya studies, the mean complete remission response is 84%. These response data require several qualifications. First, these series contain both newly diagnosed patients and relapsed patients. Second, an uncertain proportion of patients did not have the 15;17 translocation by cytogenetics or molecular testing. Nonetheless, the initial response to all-*trans*-RA in patients documented by cytogenetic or molecular analysis to have the fusion PML/ RAR-α is very high - very close to 100% of evaluable cases - and *de novo* resistance is exceptional.

The time to achieve complete remission has varied, ranging from 1 to 3 months in most series. The median time to remission was 44 days in the Shanghai series [102] and 38 days in the New York series [103]. The perception that time to remission is longer with all-*trans* RA

Table 1. Summary of clinical trials using all-*trans* retinoic acid as a single agent for remission induction treatment in acute promyelocytic leukaemia (both newly diagnosed patients and patients previously treated with combination chemotherapy are included)

Site	No. pts.	No. in CR	% CR	References
Shanghai	400	340	85%	Sun et al. 1992 [102] Huang et al. 1988 [96]
Paris	31	23	74%	Castaigne et al. 1989 [97]
New York	79	68	86%	Warrell et al. 1991 [98] Warrell et al. 1994 [101]
Suzhou	50	47	94%	Chen et al. 1991 [99]
Nagoya	26	18	70%	Ohno et al. 1992 [100]

than with chemotherapy is incorrect given the number of chemotherapy-treated patients who require more than one course of induction therapy [1,2,104].

Predictiveness of Clinical Response

Both the Chinese and French groups have observed that the *in vitro* response to all-*trans* RA is highly correlated with clinical effectiveness [92,96]. In these studies, suspensions of leukaemic cells aspirated from bone marrow were cultured in the presence of all-*trans* RA at various concentrations (usually 10^{-6} or 10^{-7} M). Practically, however, clinical exigencies often dictate the choice of treatment before obtaining culture results. Moreover, several groups have noted that relapsing patients may retain *in vitro* sensitivity while remaining clinically resistant [99,105].

The initial clinical response to all-*trans* RA is most closely correlated with the presence of the 15;17 translocation as assessed by conventional cytogenetics or by molecular assay using probes for RAR-α mRNA on Northern blot analysis [18-20,92,106,107] or reverse transcriptase-polymerase chain reaction (RT-PCR) assays with specific primers [108-113]. Each of these tests varies in its sensitivity and specificity, and proper interpretation of the laboratory result is critical. A cytogenetic result that indicates the presence of the t(15;17) is pathognomonic for APL, is associated with molecular rearrangement of the RAR-α receptor, and is highly correlated with the clinical response to all-*trans* RA. A "negative" result is problematic. Some patients who have had equivocal morphologic characteristics and reportedly normal karyotypes have shown typical rearrangements of RAR-α by molecular testing, and virtually all clinically evaluable patients have subsequently responded to all-*trans* RA [101,106,109,113]. By contrast, patients who are negative by RT-PCR for the PML/RAR-α fusion do not exhibit t(15;17) by cytogenetics, and none of these patients has responded clinically [106]. Other translocations involving RAR-α have recently been described (such as PLZF/RAR-α), but they appear to be quite uncommon [41,114]. These data argue strongly for a new molecular definition of the disease rather than distinctions based on morphology, immunophenotype, or clinical manifestations.

Duration of Remission

While *de novo* resistance to all-*trans* RA in a patient with a molecular diagnosis of APL is distinctly unusual, all investigators have observed that remissions induced and maintained by all-*trans* RA are transient; however, the actual number of patients maintained solely on all-*trans* RA is quite small. The median duration of remission in the New York series was 3.5 months, ranging from 1 to 23 months [101,103]. Remissions in other series are of similar duration, and very few patients treated only with

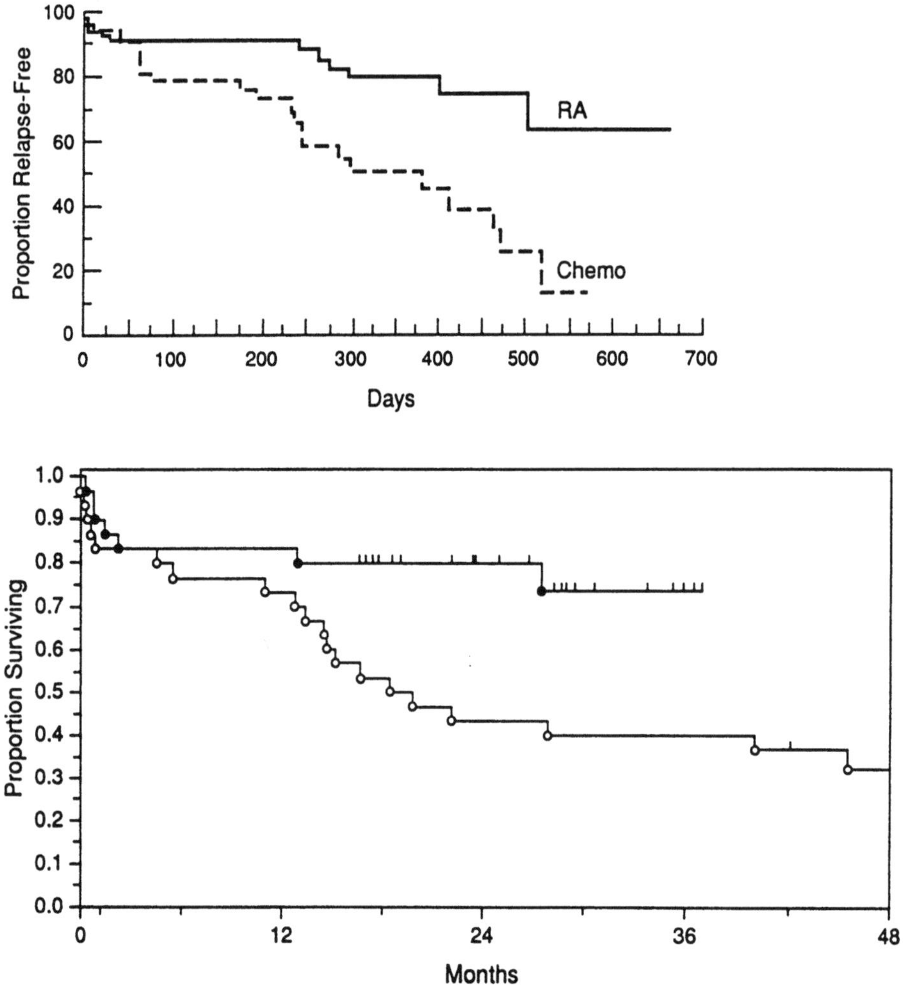

Fig. 5.
Top panel: increase in relapse-free survival in APL patients induced with all-*trans* retinoic acid followed by chemotherapy consolidation in the European randomised trial.
Redrawn from [116]
Bottom panel: increase in overall survival in APL patients induced with all-*trans* retinoic acid in the New York study.
Reprinted with permission from [101]

all-*trans* RA remain in remission longer than 1 year [96,97,99,102,103].

There is now substantial evidence from 3 clinical trials - the French pilot [115], the New York study [101,103] (both compared to historical controls), and the European randomised study [116] (compared to concurrent controls) - that an approach which combines induction with all-*trans* RA followed by standard consolidation chemotherapy yields a significant increase in relapse-free and overall survival compared to the use of chemotherapy alone (Fig. 5). As yet, no benefit has been demonstrated for the use of all-*trans* RA as maintenance, although this approach is currently being tested in both Europe and the U.S. Generally, patients who relapse while taking all-*trans* RA cannot be reinduced into remission by further treatment with all-*trans* RA [99,101] although there seems to be no increase in resistance to conventional chemotherapy.

Acquired Resistance

Given the relatively brief duration of remission, acquired resistance to all-*trans* RA could theoretically result from genetic or epigenetic causes (see [117] for review). While acquired retinoid resistance in myeloid cell lines (HL60 and NB4) has been associated with a point mutation in RAR-α [118] or altered expression of PML/RAR-α protein [45], clinical specimens have not revealed such mutations at the time of relapse as compared with pretreatment [105].

Relapse and acquired resistance to all-*trans* RA may in part be explained by its clinical pharmacology. Following a single oral dose, peak plasma drug concentrations are achieved within 1 to 2 hours; however, the drug rapidly disappears from plasma with a half-life of approximately 40 minutes [119,120]. Unexpectedly, continuous daily treatment with all-*trans* RA is associated with a progressive decrease in plasma drug concentrations [105]. Mechanisms for accelerated clearance include induction of cytochrome-P450 oxidative enzymes [105], an increase in oxidative cofactors [121, 122], and increased expression of cellular retinoic acid binding proteins (CRABP) [123, 124]. These somewhat redundant biological mechanisms function cooperatively to modulate intracellular retinoid concentrations. This reduction in plasma drug levels has been correlated with relapse and clinical resistance [105], although the association naturally does not establish the phenomenon as causal. These data do, however, suggest that clinical failure might in part be due to an inability to sustain effective "cytodifferentiating" concentrations *in vivo* during prolonged administration. This distinctive pharmacology also suggests that this agent, as compared with other potentially effective retinoids, might not be useful as "maintenance" therapy in APL.

Mechanism of Action

At the cellular level, considerable data indicate that induction of remission by all-*trans* RA is associated with differentiation of immature neoplastic cells into mature granulocytes, followed by the emergence of normal haematopoietic cells as the patient achieves remission [96-98,125,126]. Data that support this mechanism include the absence of bone marrow hypoplasia during induction, the appearance of immunophenotypically unique "intermediate cells" that co-express mature and immature cell surface antigens (indicating their derivation from the malignant clone) [98], and persistence in morphologically mature granulocytes of both Auer rods and the 15;17 chromosomal translocation until a late stage of induction [98,125]. As yet, there is no convincing evidence for a high frequency of clonal remissions in APL [127] (i.e. that a substantial proportion of phenotypically normal cells persistently carry the t[15;17] during remission). The ultimate mechanism whereby the visible population of malignant cells is eliminated is unclear. After inducing irreversible commitment to differentiation, all-*trans* RA may initiate programmed cell death (apoptosis) in the maturing cells [128]. A transient decrease in the peripheral blood leukocyte count consistently occurs late in the treatment course (3 to 4 weeks) in patients who are otherwise responding well [103]. Conceivably, this phenomenon represents final elimination of a large number of neoplastic cells followed by delayed regrowth of normal haematopoietic elements.

Treatment with retinoic acid appears to act on at least 2 stages of myeloid cell development. The maturation arrest in non-proliferating promyelocytes is obviously overcome; however, the drug must also act on earlier neoplastic progenitor cells that have retained a capacity for self-renewal but that are nonetheless already committed along a myeloid differentiation pathway. (One might also infer the existence of an earlier leukaemic progenitor pool that is RA insensitive). *In vitro*, mitosis is not required to observe differentiating effects in cell lines such as NB4 [129] or HL-60 [48,54]. Clinically, however, a relatively consistent pattern of peripheral blood leukocytosis is observed in most patients undergoing induction. It is unclear whether this phenomenon represents a transient increase in leukaemic cell survival, "release" from the bone marrow (as seen after the administration of certain colony-stimulating factors), or one or more cycles of mitosis by a cell population still capable of self-renewal prior to its maturation to a stage that is incapable of further replication.

At the molecular level, the effects of all-*trans* RA are less clear. It seems counter-intuitive that a mutation that leads to the expression of a defective receptor should confer spectacular clinical sensitivity to one of its ligands. Assuming that the primary defect is a dominant negative interference with the retinoic acid signal transduction system as suggested above, it is possible that at higher intranuclear concentrations of RA, the normal retinoid receptors would simply out-compete the aberrant PML/ RAR-α. This hypothesis is supported by observations that RXR receptors are activated only at high cytodifferentiating concentrations of retinoic acid, and that all-*trans* RA increases the expression of normal RAR-α receptors in many normal cells, including promyelocytes [130, 131].

Treatment Recommendations in APL

When employed in correctly diagnosed patients, all-*trans* RA has proven to be the most effective single agent for the treatment of any type of acute leukaemia. If the "retinoic acid syndrome" is absent (for a discussion of this and other adverse reactions, see the chapter "Clinical Toxicology of the Retinoids" in this volume), the drug is quite safe and relatively well tolerated. These characteristics notwithstanding, two critical questions are unresolved: first, what are the optimal means of maximising safety regarding leukocytosis, retinoic acid syndrome, and the haemostatic disorder of APL; second, what is the proper role of this drug in overall patient management (i.e., alone or in combination; as initial treatment or as maintenance)?

Obviously, the drug should be made available to patients who are resistant to conventional chemotherapy and to patients who have relapsed from standard treatment. Moreover, many specialists now believe that this agent represents first-line therapy for all newly diagnosed patients as well. As previously noted, 3 large and well conducted studies have shown superior remission duration and overall survival in patients induced with this drug compared with conventional chemotherapy [101,115, 116]. While preliminary data suggest that clinical response can be predicted by *in vitro* cell culture data, molecular assays for the aberrant retinoid receptor are most useful. Until these tests become widely available, it is reasonable to treat patients if they fulfill morphologic diagnostic criteria until the cytogenetic or molecular result is known.

At present, all-*trans* RA is recommended only for the induction of remission. Long-term therapy without additional chemotherapy is associated with relapse and resistance to subsequent treatment. Patients who achieve complete remission with all-*trans* RA should receive additional chemotherapy - preferably anthracycline-based - as "consolidation". For previously untreated patients, most groups discontinue the drug after achieving remission and then administer 3 cycles of anthracycline/ cytosine arabinoside combination chemotherapy [101,115,116]. As yet, there is no advantage to combining long-term all-*trans* RA treatment with chemotherapy. No consensus regarding the management of leukocytosis has yet emerged; investigative groups have variously favoured prevention using full-dose chemotherapy or no specific therapy for the leukocytosis and dexamethasone treatment at the earliest appearance of respiratory distress. Since the drug almost never induces rapid cell lysis, the administration of vigorous parenteral hydration and allopurinol to prevent consequences of tumour lysis are generally not indicated. Since many patients with incipient features of the "retinoic acid syndrome" appear to retain fluids even after steroid treatment, intravenous fluids should ideally be minimised to avoid fluid overload.

In addition to an increase in the peripheral blood leukocyte count, resolution of the coagulopathy is frequently the first sign of response to all-*trans* RA; however, tests for coagulation function (including fibrinogen, fibrin degradation products, and D-dimers) should be monitored periodically until normal. Occasionally, DIC can worsen as the terminally differentiated cells are eliminated. The management of the haemorrhagic diathesis is similar to that recommended by Tallman and Kwaan [70]. Patients with evidence of DIC should receive transfusions of platelets and fresh frozen plasma to maintain the platelet count ≥ 50,000 cells/µl and fibrinogen ≥ 100 mg/dl. Heparin is reserved for patients with marked or persistent elevation of fibrin degradation products or thrombosis [8]. Fibrinolytic inhibitors such as ε-aminocaproic acid are currently being used in cases with incipient or life-threatening retinal or intracranial haemorrhage, with or without low molecular weight heparin (enoxaparine). Treatment outside the hospital can be recommended for afebrile patients who have no requirement for platelet transfusions; however, such patients should be seen at least twice per week until complete remission has been achieved. In addition, full supportive care (antibiotics, corticosteroids and blood products) must be available on an emergency basis if needed.

Assessment of Minimal Residual Disease in APL

The presence of PML/RAR-α fusion transcripts detectable by RT/PCR has yielded a specific test for a disease that is tightly correlated with clinical responsiveness to all-*trans* RA. Since patients in first remission from APL historically have a high risk for relapse, several groups have explored the use of RT-PCR as a means of detecting minimal residual disease [32,109-113]. For the first time in any type of acute myelocytic leukaemia, these studies have enabled a real-time determination of the effects of post-remission treatments (e.g. maintenance chemotherapy, bone marrow transplantation and monoclonal antibodies). In haematological cancers, PCR technology has been used to evaluate persistence of *bcr/abl* in patients with chronic myelocytic leukaemia following bone marrow transplantation. It appears that tests for *bcr/abl* may remain positive for up to 1 year after transplantation without risk of clinical relapse [132]. At least one other type of acute myeloid leukaemia is associated with extended persistence of the RT-PCR signal in remission [113]. However, most patients with APL convert their RT-PCR signal for PML/RAR-α to negative after receiving chemotherapy consolidation [108]. More than any other finding, these data suggest that ongoing differentiation (or "clonal remissions") is not a feature of the illness, a somewhat surprising result given the natural history and response to differentiation therapy previously described.

Currently, most groups are following APL patients in remission with serial RT-PCR testing. In New York, patients are tested after each of 3 cycles of consolidation chemotherapy, then every 3 months for the first year in remission, and then at 6-month intervals for the next 2 years. It has become quite clear that a positive RT-PCR test for PML/RAR-α equates with the presence of active disease, and that a patient in otherwise "complete" remission who converts a previously negative test to positive will go on to relapse. Therefore, these patients should be considered candidates for further treatment such as bone marrow transplantation. The implications of a single negative test are doubtful; however, serially negative tests in remission have been associated with extended survival [108-113].

Summary

One of the most striking recent advances in cancer research is the conclusive documentation of differentiation as a practical and consistently effective method of treating human cancer. All-*trans* RA clearly has certain undesirable pharmacokinetic properties; however, these problems might be overcome by alternative retinoids such as 9-*cis* RA that are equally active against APL *in vitro* [133]. In addition to retinoids that selectively activate RAR or RXR receptors [134-136], other ligands of the steroid/thyroid receptor superfamily such as vitamin D_3, glucocorticoids, and sex steroids also have cytodifferentiating actions in model systems [137,138]. Therefore, it is a major objective of current research to examine interactions of these pathways in an effort to identify synergistically active combinations of these and other compounds in order to maximally exploit both this concept and induced programmed cell death as treatments for other neoplastic diseases.

Acknowledgement

This work was supported in part by grants FD-R-000764 from the Orphan Products Division, U.S. Food and Drug Administration; by CA-57645 from the U.S. National Cancer Institute; by the Fondation de France, ARC, and by the LNCC.

REFERENCES

1 Stone RM and Mayer RJ: The unique aspects of acute promyelocytic leukemia. J Clin Oncol 1990 (8):1913-1921
2 Mayer RJ, Schiffer CA, Peterson BP et al: Intensive postremission therapy in adults with acute nonlymphocytic leukemia using various dose schedules of ara-C: a progress report from the CALGB. Semin Oncol 1987 (14 suppl 1):25-31
3 Hillestad LK: Acute promyelocytic leukemia. Acta Med Scand 1957:189-194
4 Marty M, Ganem G, Fisher J et al: Leucémie aigue promyelocytaire: étude retrospective de 119 malades traités par daunorubicine. Nouv Rev Fr Hematol 1978 (26):371-378
5 Kantarjian HM, Keating MJ, Walters RS et al: Acute promyelocytic leukemia: the MD Anderson Hospital experience. Am J Med 1986 (80):789-797
6 Cunningham I, Gee TS, Reich LM, Kempin SJ, Naval AN, Clarkson BD: Acute promyelocytic leukemia: treatment results during a decade at Memorial Hospital. Blood 1989 (73):1116-1122
7 Sanz MA, Jarque I, Martin G et al: Acute promyelocytic leukemia: therapy results and prognostic factors. Cancer 1988 (61):7-13
8 Rodeghiero F, Avvisati G, Castaman G, Barbui T, Mandelli F: Early deaths and antihemorrhagic treatments in acute promyelocytic leukemia. A GIMEMA retrospective study in 268 consecutive patients. Blood 1990 (75):2112-2117
9 Cordonnier C, Vernant JP, Brun B et al: Acute promyelocytic leukemia in 57 previously untreated patients. Cancer 1985 (5)5:18-24
10 Gralnick HR and Sultan C: Acute promyelocytic leukemia: haemorrhagic manifestation and morphologic criteria. Br J Haematol 1975 (29):373-376
11 Jones ME and Saleem A: Acute promyelocytic leukemia: a review of the literature. Am J Med 1978 (65):673-677
12 Golomb HM, Rowley J, Vardiman J et al: Partial deletion of long arm of chromosome 17: a specific abnormality in acute promyelocytic leukemia? Arch Int Med 1976 (136):825-828
13 Rowley JD, Golomb HM, Dougherty C: 15/17 translocation: a consistent chromosomal change in acute promyelocytic leukemia. Lancet 1977 (1): 549-550
14 Larson RA, Kondo K, Vardiman JW, Butler AE, Golomb HM, Rowley JD: Evidence for a 15;17 translocation in every patient with acute promyelocytic leukemia. Am J Med 1984 (76):827-841
15 Mattei MG, Petkovich M, Mattei JF, Brand N, Chambon, P: Mapping of the human retinoic acid receptor to the q21 band of chromosome 17. Hum Genet 1988 (80):186-188
16 Chomienne C, Ballerini P, Balitrand N et al: The retinoic acid receptor α gene is rearranged in retinoic-acid sensitive promyelocytic leukemia. Leukemia 1990 (4):802-807
18 Longo L, Pandolfi PP, Biondi A et al: Rearrangement and aberrant expression of the retinoic acid receptor α in acute promyelocytic leukemia. J Exp Med 1990 (72):1571-1575
19 Chang KS, Trujillo JM, Ogura T et al: Rearrangement of the retinoic acid receptor gene in acute promyelocytic leukemia. Leukemia 1991 (5):200-204
20 Chen Z, Chen SJ, Tong JH et al: The retinoic acid receptor α gene is frequently disrupted in its 5' part in Chinese patients with acute promyelocytic leukemia. Leukemia 1990 (5):288-292
21 Borrow J, Goddard AD, Sheer D, Solomon E: Molecular analysis of acute promyelocytic leukemia breakpoint cluster region on chromosome 17. Science 1990 (249):1577-1580
22 de Thé H, Chomienne C, Lanotte M, Degos L, Dejean A: The t(15;17) translocation of acute promyelocytic leukaemia fuses the retinoic acid receptor α gene to a novel transcribed locus. Nature 1990 (347):558-561
23 Alcalay M, Zangrilli D, Paolo P et al: Translocation breakpoint of acute promyelocytic leukemia lies within the retinoic acid receptor α locus. Proc Natl Acad Sci (USA) 1991 (88):1977-1981
24 Lemmons R, Eilender D, Waldmann R et al: Cloning and characterization of the t(15,17) translocation breakpoint region in acute promyelocytic leukemia. Genes Chromosomes Cancer 1990 (2):79-87
25 Goddard A, Borrow J, Freemont P et al: Characterisation of a zinc finger gene disrupted by the t(15,17) translocation in acute promyelocytic leukemia. Science 1991 (254):1371-1374
27 Kakizuka A, Miller WH Jr, Umesono K et al: Chromosomal translocation t(15,17) in human acute promyelocytic leukemia fuses RAR-α with a novel putative transcription factor PML. Cell 1991 (66):663-674
28 de Thé H, Lavau C, Marchio A et al: The PML/RAR-α fusion mRNA generated by the t(15,17) translocation encodes a functionally altered retinoic acid receptor. Cell 1991 (66):675-684
29 Pandolfi PP, Grignani F, Alcalay M et al: Structure and origin of the acute promyelocytic leukemia *myl*/RAR-α cDNA and characterization of its retinoid binding and transactivation properties. Oncogene 1991 (6):1285-1292
30 Kastner P, Perez A, Lutz Y et al: Structure, localization and transcriptional properties of two classes of retinoic acid receptor α fusion proteins in acute promyelocytic leukemia: structural similarities with a new family of oncoproteins. EMBO J 1992 (11):629-642
31 Tong JH, Dong S, Geng JP et al: Molecular rearrangements of the *myl* gene in acute promyelocytic leukemia define a breakpoint cluster region as well as some molecular variants. Oncogene 1992 (7):311-316
32 Chang KS, Lu J, Trujillo JM et al: The t(15;17) translocation in acute promyelocytic leukemia clusters in two different sites of the *myl* gene: targets for the detection of minimal residual disease by the polymerase chain reaction. Blood 1992 (79):544-558
33 Solomon E, Borrow J, Goddard AD: Chromosome aberrations and cancer. Science 1991 (254):1153-1160

34 Lewin B: Oncogenic changes by regulatory changes in transcription factors. Cell 1992 (64): 303-312

35 Clarkson B: Acute promyelocytic leukemia: the promise and the paradox. Cancer Cells 1991 (3): 211-219

36 Lovering R, Hanson IM, Borden KLB et al: Identification and preliminary charaterization of a protein motif related to the zinc finger. Proc Natl Acad Sci (USA) 1993 (90):2112-2116

37 Reddy B, Etkin L, Freemont P: A novel zinc finger coiled-coil domain in a family of nuclear proteins. Trends Biochem Sci 1992 (17):344-345

38 Daniel MT, Koken M, Romagne O et al: PML protein expression in hematopoietic and APL cells. Blood 1993 (82):1858-1867

39 Koken M, Puvion F, Guillemin MC et al: The t(15;17) translocation alters a nuclear body in a RA-reversible fashion. EMBO J 1994 (14):1073-1083

40 Dyck J, Maul G, Miller W, Chen D, Kakizuka A, Evans R: A novel macromolecular structure is a target of the promyelocyte-retinoic acid receptor oncoprotein. Cell 1994 (76):333-343

41 Chen S, Brand N, Chen A et al: Fusion between a novel kruppel-like finger gene and the retinoic acid receptor α locus due to a variant t(11;17) translocation associated with acute promyelocytic leukemia. EMBO J 1993 (12):1161-1167

42 Nagpal S, Saunders M, Kastner P et al: Promoter context and response element-dependent specificity of the transcriptional activation and modulating functions of retinoic acid receptors. Cell 1992 (70):1007-1019

43 Pandolfi PP, Alcalay M, Fagioli M et al: Genomic variability and alternative splicing generate multiple PML/RARα transcripts that encode aberrant PML proteins and PML/RARA isoforms in acute promyelocytic leukemias. EMBO J 1992 (11):1397-1407

44 Perez A, Kastner P, Sethi S, Reibel C, Chambon P: PML/RAR-α homodimers, distinct DNA-binding properties and heterodimeric interactions with RXRs. EMBO J 1993 (12):3171-3182

45 Grignani F, Ferrucci PF, Testa U et al: The acute promyelocytic leukemia-specific PML/RARα fusion protein inhibits differentation and promotes survival of myeloid precursor cells. Cell 1993 (74): 423-431

46 Tobler A, Dawson MI, Koeffler HP: Retinoids: structure-function relationship in normal and leukemic hematopoiesis. J Clin Invest 1986 (78): 303-309

47 Douer D and Koeffler HP: Retinoic acid enhances colony stimulating factor-induced clonal growth of normal human myeloid progenitor cells in vitro. Exp Cell Res 1982 (138):193-201

48 Breitman TR, Selonick SE, Collins SJ: Induction of differentiation of the human promyelocytic leukemia cell line (HL60) by retinoic acid. Proc Natl Acad Sci (USA) 1980 (77):2936-2940

49 Shroeder C, Gibson L, Zenke M, Beug H: Modulation of normal erythroid differentiation by the endogenous thyroid and retinoid acid receptors: possible targets for v-*erb* a oncogene action. Oncogene 1992 (7):217-227

50 Collins SJ, Robertson KA, Mueller L: Retinoic acid-induced granulocytic differentiation of HL-60 myeloid leukemia cells is mediated directly through the retinoic acid receptor (RAR-α). Mol Cell Biol 1990 (10):2154-2163

52 Tsai S, Bartelmez S, Heyman R, Damm K, Evans R, Collins S: A mutated retinoic acid receptor α exhibiting dominant negative activity alters the lineage development of a multi-potent hematopoietic cell line. Genes Devel 1992 (6):2258-2269

52 Tsai S and Collins S: A dominant negative retinoic acid receptor blocks neutrophil differentiation at the promyelocytic stage. Proc Natl Acad Sci (USA) 1993 (90):7153-7157

53 Sharif M and Privalsky M: v-erbA oncogene function in neoplasia correlates with its ability to repress RAR action. Cell 1991 (66):885-893

54 Rousselot P, Hardas B, Castaigne S et al: The PML-RAR gene product of the t(15;17) translocation inhibits retinoic acid induced granulocytic differentiation. Oncogene 1994 (in press)

55 Ascoli CA and Maul GG: Identification of a novel nuclear domain. J Cell Biol 1991 (112):785-795

60 de Thé G, Rivière M, Bernhard W: Bull Cancer 1960 (47):570-584

61 Szostecki C, Guldner HH, Netter HJ, Will H: Isolation and characterisation of a cDNA encoding a human nuclear antigen predominantly recognized by auto antibodies of patients with primary billiary cirrhosis. J Immunol 1990 (145):4338-4347

62 Eilers M, Picard D, Yamwnoto K, Bishop M: Chimaeras of the *myc* oncoprotein and the steroid receptors cause hormone-dependent transformation of cells. Nature 1989 (340):66-68

63 Mangelsdorf D and Evans R: The retinoid receptor network. In: McKnight S and Yamamoto K (eds) Transcriptional Regulation. Cold Spring Harbor Press, Cold Spring Harbor, NY. Vol. 2, pp 1137-1167

66 Ganem G, Fischer J, Marty M et al: Prognostic factors in acute promyelocytic leukemia (APL): a retrospective study of 101 patients treated by daunorubicin containing remission induction regimen. Blood 1983 (63 suppl):171a

67 Ventura GJ, Hester JP, Dixon DO, Khorana S, Keating MJ: Analysis of risk factors for fatal hemorrhage during induction therapy of patients with acute promyelocytic leukemia. Hematol Pathol 1989 (3):23-28

68 Berman E, Little C, Kher U et al: Prognostic analysis of patients with acute promyelocytic leukemia (APL). Blood 1991 (78 suppl):43a

69 Thomas X, Archimbaud E, Treille-Ritouet, Fiere D: Prognostic factors in acute promyelocytic leukemia: a retrospective study of 67 cases. Leuk Lymphoma 1991 (4):249-256

70 Tallman MS and Kwaan HC: Reassessing the hemostatic disorder associated with acute promyelocytic leukemia. Blood 1992 (79):543-553

71 Gouault-Heilmann M, Chardon E, Sultan C, Josso F: The procoagulant factor of leukemic promyelocytes: demonstration of immunologic cross reactivity with human brain tissue factor. Br J Haematol 1975 (30):151-158

72 Kubota T, Andoh K, Sadakata H, Tanaka H, Koboyashi N: Tissue factor released from leukemic cells. Thromb Haemost 1991 (65):59-63
73 Bauer KA and Rosenberg RD: Thrombin generation in acute promyelocytic leukemia. Blood 1984 (64): 791-796
73 Bennett B, Booth A, Croll A, Dawson AA: The bleeding disorder in acute promyelocytic leukaemia: fibrinolysis due to u-PA rather than defibrination. Br J Haematol 1989 (71):511-517
74 Wilson EL, Jacobs P, Dowdle EB: The secretion of plasminogen activators by human myeloid leukemic cells in vitro. Blood 1983 (61):568-574
76 Francis RB and Seyfert U: Tissue plasminogen activator antigen and activity in disseminated intravascular coagulation. Clinicopathologic correlations. J Lab Clin Med 1987 (110):541-547
77 Sterrenberg L, Haak HL, Brommer EJP, Nieuwenhuizen W: Evidence of fibrinogen breakdown by leukocyte enzymes in a patient with acute promyelocytic leukemia. Haemostasis 1985 (15):126-133
78 Saito M, Asakura H, Uotani C, Jokaji H, Kumabashiri I, Matsuda T: Quantitative estimation of elastase-α-1 proteinase inhibitor (E-αPI) complex in leukemia: marked elevation in cases of acute promyelocytic leukemia. Thromb Res 1989 (53):163-171
79 Avvisati G, ten Cate JW, Sturk A, Lamping R, Petti MC, Mandelli F: Acquired α-2-antiplasmin deficiency in acute promyelocytic leukaemia. Br J Haematol 1988 (70):43-48
80 Brower NS and Harpel PC: Proteolytic cleavage and inactivation of α-2 plasmin inhibitor and C1 inactivator by human polymorphonuclear leukocyte elastase. J Biol Chem 1982 (257):9849-9854
81 Sakata Y, Murakami T, Noro A, Mori K, Matsuda M: The specific activity of plasminogen activator inhibitor-1 in disseminated intravascular coagulation with acute promyelocytic leukemia. Blood 1991 (77):1949-1957
82 Schwartz BS, Williams EC, Conlan MG, Mosher DF: Epsilon-aminocaproic acid in the treatment of patients with acute promyelocytic leukemia and acquired α-2-plasmin inhibitor. Ann Intern Med 1986 (105):873-877
83 Scrobohaci ML, Dombret H, Ghorra P et al: Disseminated intravascular coagulation (DIC) and/or primary fibrinolysis in acute promyelocytic leukemia, effect of all-*trans* retinoic acid treatment. Blood 1991 (78 suppl):48a
84 Avvisati G, Mandelli F, Petti MC et al: Idarubicin as a single agent for remission induction of previously untreated acute promyelocytic leukemia: a pilot study of the Italian cooperative group (GIMEMA). Eur J Haematol 1990 (44):257-260
85 Stone RM, Maguire M, Goldberg MA, Antin JH, Rosenthal DS, Mayer RJ: Complete remission in acute promyelocytic leukemia despite persistance of abnormal bone marrow promyelocytes during induction therapy: experience in 34 patients. Blood 1988 (71):690-696
86 Head DR, Kopecky K, Hewlett J et al: Survival with cytotoxic therapy in acute promyelocytic leukemia: a SWOG report. Blood 1991 (78 suppl):268a
87 Kantarjian H, Keating M, Walters R et al: Role of maintenance chemotherapy in acute promyelocytic leukemia. Cancer 1987 (59):1258-1263
88 Flynn PJ, Miller WJ, Weisdorf DJ, Arthur DC, Brunning R, Branda RF: Retinoic acid treatment of acute promyelocytic leukemia: in vitro and in vivo observations. Blood 1983 (62):1211-1217
89 Daenen S, Vellenga E, van Dobbenburgh OA, Halie MR: Retinoic acid as antileukemic therapy in a patient with acute promyelocytic leukemia and Aspergillus pneumonia. Blood 1986 (67):559-561
90 Fontana JA, Rogers JS, Durham JP: The role of 13-*cis* retinoic acid in the remission induction of a patient with acute promyelocytic leukemia. Cancer 1989 (57):209-217
91 Wijermans PW, Rebel VI, Ossenkoppele GJ, Huijens PC, Langenhuijsen MMAC: Combined procoagulant activity and proteolytic activity of acute promyelocytic leukemic cells: reversal of the bleeding disorder by cell differentiation. Blood 1989 (73):800-805
92 Chomienne C, Ballerini P, Balitrand N et al: All-*trans* retinoic acid in acute promyelocytic leukemias. II. In vitro studies: structure-function relationship. Blood 1990 (76):1710-1717
93 Degos L, Chomienne C, Daniel MT et al: Treatment of first relapse in acute promyelocytic leukemia with all-*trans* retinoic acid. Lancet 1990 (336): 1440-1441
94 Runde V, Aul C, Sudhoft T, Heyll A, Schneider W: Retinoic acid in the treatment of acute promyelocytic leukemia: inefficacy of the 13-*cis* isomer and induction of complete remission by the all-*trans* isomer complicated by thromboembolic events. Ann Hematol 1992 (64):270-272
95 Huang ME, Ye YC, Chen SR et al: All-*trans* retinoic acid with or without low dose cytosine arabinoside in acute promyelocytic leukemia - Report of 6 cases. Chin Med J 1987 (100):949-953
96 Huang ME, Ye YC, Chen SR et al: Use of all-*trans* retinoic acid in the treatment of acute promyelocytic leukemia. Blood 1988 (72):567-572
97 Castaigne S, Chomienne C, Daniel MT et al: All-trans retinoic acid as a differentiation therapy for acute promyelocytic leukemia: I. clinical results. Blood 1990 (76):1704-1709
98 Warrell RP Jr, Frankel SR, Miller WH Jr et al: Differentiation therapy of acute promyelocytic leukemia with tretinoin (all-*trans* retinoic acid). N Engl J Med 1991 (324):1385-1393
99 Chen ZX, Xue YQ, Zhang RI et al: A clinical and experimental study on all-*trans* retinoic acid-treated acute promyelocytic leukemia patients. Blood 1991 (78):1413-1419
100 Ohno R, Yoshida H, Naoe T et al: All-*trans* retinoic acid (ATRA) as a differentiation therapy for refractory acute promyelocytic leukemia (APL). Proc Am Assoc Cancer Res 1992 (33):234
101 Warrell RP Jr, Maslak P, Eardley A, Heller G, Miller WH, Frankel SR: Treatment of acute promyelocytic leukemia with all-*trans* retinoic acid: an update of the New York experience. Leukemia 1994 (8):929-933
102 Sun GL, Huang YG, Chang XF, Jiang GS, Zhang T: Clinial study on all-*trans* retinoic acid in treatment

of 544 cases of acute promyelocytic leukemia. Chin J Hematol 1992 (13):135-137
103 Frankel SR, Eardley A, Heller G et al: All-*trans* retinoic acid for acute promyelocytic leukemia: results of the New York study. Ann Intern Med 1994 (120):278-286
104 Eardley AM, Heller G, Warrell RP Jr: Morbidity and costs of remission induction therapy with all-*trans* retinoic acid compared with standard chemotherapy in acute promyelocytic leukemia. Leukemia 1994 (8):934-939
105 Muindi J, Frankel SR, Miller WH et al: Continuous treatment with all-*trans* retinoic acid results in a progressive decrease in plasma concentrations: implications for relapse and "resistance" in acute promyelocytic leukemia. Blood 1992 (79):299-303
106 Miller WH Jr, Levine K, DeBlasio A, Frankel SR, Dmitrovsky E, Warrell RP Jr: Detection of minimal residual disease in acute promyelocytic leukemia by reverse transcription polymerase chain reaction assay for the PML/RAR-α fusion mRNA. Blood 1993 (82):1689-1694
107 Lo Coco F, Avvisati G, Diverio D et al: Molecular evaluation of response to all-*trans* retinoic acid therapy in patients with acute promyelocytic leukemia. Blood 1991 (77):1657-1659
108 Miller WH Jr, Jakubowski A, Warrell RP Jr: 9-*cis* retinoic acid (RA), the RXR ligand, is an effective cytodifferentiating agent for acute promyelocytic leukemia (APL) cells. Blood 1992 (80 suppl):108a
109 Biondi A, Rambaldi A, Pandolfi PP, et al. Molecular monitoring of the *myl*/RAR-a fusion gene in acute promyelocytic leukemia by polymerase chain reaction. Blood 1992 (80):492-497
110 Castaigne S, Balitrand N, de Thé H, Dejean A, Degos L, Chomienne C: A PML/retinoic acid receptor α fusion transcript is constantly detected by RNA-based polymerase chain reaction in acute promyelocytic leukemia. Blood 1992 (79):3110-3115
111 Chen SJ, Chen Z, Chen A et al: Occurrence of distinct PML/RAR α fusion gene isoforms in patients with acute promyelocytic leukemia detected by the polymerase chain reaction. Oncogene 1992 (7):1223-1232
112 Borrow J, Goddard A, Gibbons B et al: Diagnosis of acute promyelocytic leukaemia by RT-PCR: detection of PML/RAR-α and RAR-α/PML fusion transcripts. Br J Haematol 1992 (82):529-540
113 Lo Coco F, Diverio D, Pandolfi PP et al: Molecular evaluation of residual disease as a predictor of relapse in acute promyelocytic leukaemia. Lancet 1992 (340):1437-1438
114 Chen Z, Guidez F, Rousselot P et al: PLZF-RARα fusion proteins generated from the variant t(11;17) (q23;q21) translocation in acute promyelocytic leukemia inhibit ligand-dependent transactivation of wild-type retinoic acid receptors. Proc Natl Acad Sci (USA) 1994 (91):1178-1182
115 Fenaux P, Le Deley MC, Castaigne S et al: Effect of all-*trans* retinoic acid in newly diagnosed acute promyelocytic leukemia; results of a multicenter randomized trial. Blood 1993 (82):3241-3249
116 Fenaux P, Castaigne S, Dombret H et al: All-*trans* retinoic acid followed by intensive chemotherapy gives a high complete remission rate and may prolong remissions in newly diagnosed acute promyelocytic leukemia: a pilot study on 26 cases. Blood 1992 (80):2176-2181
117 Warrell RP Jr, de Thé H, Wang Z-Y, Degos L: Acute promyelocytic leukemia. N Engl J Med 1993 (329):177-189
118 Robertson KA, Emami B, Collins SJ: Retinoic acid-resistant HL-60R cells harbor a point mutation in the retinoic acid receptor ligand-binding domain that confers dominant negative activity. Blood 1992 (80):1885-1889
119 Lefebvre P, Thomas G, Gourmel B et al: Pharmacokinetics of oral all-*trans* retinoic acid in patients with acute promyelocytic leukemia. Leukemia 1991 (5):1054-1058
120 Muindi J, Frankel S, Huselton C et al: Clinical pharmacology of oral all-*trans* retinoic acid in patients with acute promyelocytic leukemia. Cancer Res 1992 (52):2138-2142
121 Muindi JF and Young CW: Lipid hydroperoxides greatly increase the rate of oxidative catabolism of all-*trans* retinoic acid by human cell culture microsomes genetically enriched in specified cytochrome P-450 isoforms. Cancer Res 1993 (53): 1226-1229
122 Muindi, JF Scher HI, Rigas JR, Warrell RP Jr, Young CW: Elevated plasma lipid peroxide content correlates with rapid plasma clearance of all-trans retinoic acid in patients with advanced cancer. Cancer Res 1994 (54):2125-2128
123 Cornic M, Delva L, Guidez F, Balitrand N, Degos L, Chomienne C: Induction of retinoic acid-binding protein in normal and malignant human myeloid cells by retinoic acid in acute promyelocytic leukemia patients. Cancer Res 1992 (52):3329-3334
125 Elliott S, Taylor K, White S et al: Proof of differentiative mode of action of all-*trans* retinoic acid in acute promyelocytic leukemia using X-linked clonal analysis. Blood 1992 (79):1916-1919
126 Bashford J, Szer J, Wiley JS et al: Treatment of acute promyelocytic leukemia relapsing after allogeneic bone marrow transplantation with all-*trans* retinoic acid: suppression of the leukemic clone. Br J Haematol 1991 (79):331-334
127 Fearon ER, Burke PJ, Schiffer CA et al: Differentiation of leukemia cells to polymorphonuclear leukocytes in patients with acute nonlymphoblastic leukemia. N Engl J Med 1986 (315):15-24
128 Martin S, Bradley J, Cotter T: HL-60 cells cells induced to differentiate towards neutrophils subsequently die via apoptosis. Clin Exp Immunol 1990 (79):448-453
129 Lanotte M, Martin V, Najman S et al: NB4, a maturation inducible cell-line with t(15;17) marker isolated from a human promyelocytic leukaemia (M3). Blood 1991 (77):1080-1086
130 Chomienne C, Balitrand N, Ballerini P, Castaigne S, de The H, Degos L: All-*trans* retinoic acid modulates retinoic acid receptor-α in promyelocytic cells. J Clin Invest 1991 (88):2150-2154
131 Leroy P, Krust A, Zelent A et al: Multiple isoforms of the mouse retinoic acid receptor α are generated

by alternative splicing and differential induction by retinoic acid. EMBO J 1991 (10):59-69
132 Hughes TP, Morgan GJ, Martiat P, Goldman JM: Detection of residual leukemia after bone marrow transplant for chronic myeloid leukemia: role of polymerase chain reaction for the rearranged retinoic acid receptor-α predicts polymerase chain reaction in predicting relapse. Blood 1991 (77):874-878
133 Miller WH Jr, Warrell RP Jr, Frankel SR et al: Novel retinoic acid receptor-α transcripts in acute promyelocytic leukemia responsive to all-*trans* retinoic acid. JNCI 1990 (82):1932-1933
134 Levin A, Struenbecker L, Kazmer S, Bosakowski T, Huselton C, Allenby G, Speck J, Kratzeisen C, Rosenberger M, Lovey A, Grippo JF. 9 *cis* retinoic acid stereoisomer binds and activates the nuclear receptor RXR-α. Nature 1992 (335):359-361
135 Heyman RA, Mangelsdorf DF, Dyck JA, Stein RB, Eichele G, Evans RM: 9-*cis* retinoic acid is a high affinity ligand for the retinoid X receptor. Cell 1992 (68):397-406
136 Lehmann JM, Jong L, Fanjul A et al: Retinoids selective for retinoid X receptor response pathways. Science 1992 (258):1944-1946
137 Kizaki M, Norman AW, Bishop JE, Lin C-W, Karmakar A, Koeffler HP: 1,25-dihydroxyvitamin D_3 receptor RNA: expression in hematopoietic cells. Blood 1991 (77):1238-1247
138 Perlman K, Kutner A, Prahl J et al: 24-homologated 1,25-dihydroxyvitamin D_3 compounds: separation of calcium and cell differentiation activities. Biochemistry 1990 (29):190-196

Retinoid Therapy of Other Haematological Malignancies

David R. Parkinson [1] and Raymond P. Warrell, Jr [2]

1 Investigational Drug Branch, Division of Cancer Treatment, National Cancer Institute, Bethesda, MD 20892, U.S.A.
2 Department of Medicine, Memorial Sloan-Kettering Cancer Center, 1275 York Avenue, New York, NY 10021, U.S.A.

Retinoids appear to play an important role in the biology of the normal myeloid and lymphoid systems, and have been used in attempts at therapy in haematological premalignant states and in haematological malignancies other than acute promyelocytic syndrome.

Myelodysplastic Syndromes

Retinoids have been used extensively as therapeutic agents in the therapy of myelodysplastic syndromes (MDS), with ambiguous results. 13-*cis* RA has been the most extensively studied retinoid, often used in combination with cytosine arabinoside, vitamin D3, or interferon alpha. Phase I and II studies of 13-*cis* RA have sometimes suggested benefit for individual patients. At least 4 of 69 patients on pilot studies were reported to undergo complete haematological remissions, and in one patient this improvement was associated with the disappearance of cytogenetic abnormalities [1]. A double-blind, placebo-controlled, randomised study of 13-*cis* RA in 68 assessable patients with myelodysplastic syndrome, however, did not establish any benefit to the use of the retinoid [2]. One caution to the interpretation of this study is that a high frequency of drug toxicity was encountered, requiring dose reduction or therapy termination. Clark et al. also conducted a randomised trial comparing lower-dose 13-*cis* RA with supportive care; these investigators demonstrated a survival benefit only in a retrospectively determined subset of patients with refractory anaemia and less than 5% blasts [3,4]. The investigators suggested that in future trials different subgroups of patients with myelodysplastic syndromes should be prospectively identified for separate analysis [3,4]. Picozzi et al. reported on 15 patients with MDS treated with 13-*cis* RA; 8 of these patients experienced an increase in granulocyte counts greater than 20% [5], as predicted by *in vitro* colony assays [6].

The toxicity of long-term 13-*cis* RA has been limiting in this group of patients, and since there have been suggestions that prolonged therapy with 13-*cis* RA may result in increased response rates, Besa et al. have combined this retinoid with alpha-tocopherol in an attempt to decrease toxicity and permit more extended drug therapy in patients with myelodysplastic syndromes [7]. The response rate in the initial trial using this strategy was 26% in 45 assessable patients.

Other retinoids have also been studied in patients with MDS. Fenretinide (4-HPR) was utilised in a phase II trial, with no response among 14 assessable patients; in this trial 2 patients experienced acceleration of disease during therapy with fenretinide [8]. More recently, clinical trials of all-*trans* retinoic acid have been initiated in patients with MDS; all-*trans* RA is being used either alone or in combination with other differentiation inducing agents such as hexamethylene bisacetamide (HMBA), or haematopoietic growth factors. For example, Ganser et al. [9] have provided preliminary results of a clinical trial in MDS patients of the combination of all-*trans* retinoic acid, granulocyte colony stimulating factor (G-CSF), erythropoietin and vitamin E. Of 15 patients with either refractory anaemia, refractory with ring sideroblasts, or refractory with excess of blasts, all patients experienced an increase in absolute neutrophil count, and 7 patients an increase in erythropoiesis. Platelet counts increased in 3 patients, but in 3 patients they decreased; this decrease was correlated with a concomitant significant increase in serum TNF-alpha levels. Adverse effects encountered with this regimen included the expected mild dermatitis and cheilosis.

Non-APL Acute Myeloblastic Leukaemia

The sensitivity of M3 acute myeloblastic leukaemia (AML) to all-*trans* retinoic acid, as discussed in the chapter by de Thé et al. elsewhere in this monograph, appears to be unique [10]. *In vitro*, non-M3 AML cells are less sensitive, although this sensitivity may be increased by the use together with retinoids of other differentiating agents including haematopoietic growth factors. Although a number of studies using all-*trans* RA are ongoing, there is only limited clinical experience with retinoids in non-M3 AML. A phase II study published by the Paediatric Oncology Group described 1 complete and 2 partial responses among 41 children with AML treated with 13-*cis* RA [11]. The CR was achieved in a patient with M5 subtype, and the PRs in patients with M4 and M7 subtypes. While retinyl palmitate was used in maintenance therapy of another group of children with AML who had been induced to remission, the design of the study does not allow evaluation of the contribution of the retinoid [12]. While 13-*cis* RA was not active in a group of 12 elderly patients with AML [13], there were 2 haematological responses in patients with M2 and M4 subtypes in another study [14]. There has been limited published experience using retinoids in combination with other agents such as cytosine arabinoside or haematological growth factors [15], although laboratory studies support the use of this combination [16,17]. A recent optimistic report of a pilot study suggested that the combination of all-*trans* RA (at 45 mg/m^2/d) and low-dose cytosine arabinoside (at 20 mg/m^2 subcutaneously twice daily for 10 days) was both well tolerated and effective when used in a group of patients with relapsed or refractory AML, or in elderly patients in whom aggressive initial therapy was not indicated [18]. The combination of all-*trans* RA and G-CSF administered following initial therapy with cytosine arabinoside (200 mg/ m^2/d for 5 days) was piloted in a study at Memorial Sloan-Kettering Cancer Center involving patients with refractory/relapsed AML [19]. The rationale for this combination related to the superadditive *in vitro* maturation of patient leukaemic cells with the combination of the retinoid and the growth factor. Again, therapy was described as well tolerated. In the first 4 evaluable patients one patient achieved a complete remission. These pilot experiences demonstrate the tolerability of these combinations, and suggest that comparative trials to evaluate the value of retinoids in combination with other agents in this clinical setting may be indicated.

Juvenile Chronic Myelogenous Leukaemia

This disorder is distinguished from adult chronic myelogenous leukaemia by its onset in infancy or early childhood, its rapid course and the presence of prominent monocytosis and elevated foetal haemoglobin, along with the absence of a Philadelphia chromosome [20]. Haematopoietic progenitor cells from these patients respond to lower concentrations of granulocyte-macrophage colony stimulating factor (GM-CSF) than do normal progenitor cells [21]. Furthermore, a characteristic *in vitro* finding on bone marrow culture in these patients is the excessive proliferation of monocyte-macrophage colonies even in the absence of an exogenously added source of colony stimulating factors [22]. The spontaneous proliferative capacity is effectively blocked either by depletion of adherent cells from the culture, or by the use of neutralising antibodies specific for GM-CSF [23]. *In vitro*, addition of 13-*cis* RA to the cultures is associated with reduction of spontaneous growth of these JCML progenitor cells, apparently through a retinoid-mediated decrease in the hypersensitivity of the cells to GM-CSF [21, 24]. As predicted by the *in vitro* culture results, 13-*cis* RA appears to have activity in patients with juvenile chronic myelogenous leukaemia; the initial therapeutic results in 8 treated children who received 100 mg/m^2/d of the retinoid included 2 complete and 2 partial responses [24].

Multiple Myeloma

There is some laboratory data to justify clinical exploration of the use of retinoids in patients with multiple myeloma. Sidell et al. have demonstrated that *in vitro*, all-*trans* RA causes growth inhibition of a multiple myeloma cell line at concentrations readily achievable *in vivo*, with a half-maximal effect observed at 10 nmol/l, and maximal effects at 10 μmol/l [25]. These investigators further demonstrated that IL-6 receptors were down-regulated following the period of retinoid exposure in these myeloma cells, an important observation in the context of the earlier observations by Kawano et al. concerning the apparent autocrine growth factor activity of IL-6 in myeloma cells [26]. Despite this rationale, the initial clinical experience with all-*trans* RA is not encouraging. Vesole et al. [27] recently reported on 11 patients with refractory multiple myeloma who were treated at a dose of 50 mg/m^2 3 times daily of all-*trans* RA. There were no objective responses in this group of very heavily pretreated patients.

Mycosis Fungoides

Mycosis fungoides and the closely related Sezary syndrome represent T-lymphocyte malignancies of CD4-positive phenotype [28]. Treatment in patients who progress to disseminated disease is unsatisfactory, and several retinoids have been studied in clinical trials for their activity in this setting. Eleven of 25 (44%) largely previously treated patients attained objective responses to 13-*cis* RA administered at 1-2 mg/kg/d, with 3 of the patients achieving complete responses [29,30]. Similar results, with complete response in 21% and partial response in 46% of patients, were obtained in a clinical trial conducted by the Scandinavian Mycosis Fungoides Groups, using 13-*cis* RA at an initial dose of 2 mg/kg/d, with subsequent dose reductions to 0.2-0.5 mg/d [31]. These investigators noted clinical improvement within 2 to 4 weeks on initiation of treatment, and patients achieving complete response did so within 2 months.

A clinical trial conducted by Zachariae et al. [32] tested the combination of interferon-alpha and etretinate. As a single agent, interferon-alpha is known to be active in mycosis fungoides; the biological evidence that the combination of interferon and retinoids may have synergistic activity is reviewed in the chapter by Pastorino et al. in this monograph. In this pilot study, 4 of 7 patients responded.

Hoting and Meissner [33] reported on 6 patients with cutaneous T-cell lymphoma who were treated with an arotinoid-ethylester (Ro 13-6298); one patient achieved a complete response lasting longer than 102 weeks, and 2 other patients achieved partial responses. Using the same arotinoid, Mahrle and Thiele achieved partial responses in 3 out of 5 patients treated with Ro-6298, and in 4 of 6 patients who were treated with etretinate in combination with PUVA [34].

Recently, Kuzel et al. [35] reported on 13 patients with mycosis fungoides or the Sezary syndrome treated with all-*trans* RA at 45 mg/m^2. All patients had failed at least one previous therapeutic agent, with the group overall having received a median of 4 previous therapies. Four partial responses (31%) were noted in this group of patients, with minimal toxicity encountered.

Acknowledgement

This work was supported in part by grants to RPW: FD-R-000764 from the Orphan Products Division, U.S. Food and Drug Administration and by CA-57645 from the U.S. National Cancer Institute.

REFERENCES

1 Abrahm J, Besa E, Hyzinski M et al: Disappearance of cytogenetic abnormalities and clinical remission during therapy with 13-cis retinoic acid in a patient with myelodysplastic syndrome. Inhibition of growth of the patient's malignant monocytoid clone. Blood 1986 (67):1323-1327

2 Koeffler J, Heitjan D, Mertelsmann R et al: Randomized study of 13-cis retinoic acid versus placebo in the myelodysplastic disorders. Blood 1988 (71): 703-708

3 Clark R, Ismail S, Jacobs A et al: A randomized trial of 13-cis retinoic acid with or without cytosine arabinoside in patients with the myelodysplastic syndrome. Br J Haematol 1987 (66):77-83

4 Clark R, Lush C, Jacobs A et al: Effect of 13-cis retinoic acid on survival of patients with myelodysplastic syndrome. Lancet 1987 (1):763-765

5 Picozzi V, Swanson G, Morgan R et al: 13-cis retinoic acid treatment for myelodysplastic syndromes. J Clin Oncol 1986 (4):589-595

6 Swanson G, Picozzi V, Morgan R et al: Responses of hemopoietic precursors to 13-cis retinoic acid and 1,25 dihydroxyvitamin D3 in the myelodysplastic syndromes. Blood 1986 (67):1154-1161

7 Besa E, Abrahm J, Bartholomew M et al: Treatment with 13-cis retinoic acid in transfusion-dependent patients with myelodysplastic syndrome and decreased toxicity with addition of alpha-tocopherol. Am J Med 1990 (89):739-747

8 Garewal H, List A, Meyskens F et al: Phase II trial of fenretinide [No(4-hydroxyphenyl)retinamide] in myelodysplasia: Possible retinoid-induced disease acceleration. Leuk Res 1989 (13):339-343

9 Ganser A, Ottmann OG, Schadeck Gressel C et al: Combination therapy with all-trans retinoic acid, granulocyte colony-stimulating factor, erythropoietin and vitamin E in patients with myelodysplastic syndromes. Blood 1993 (82 suppl 1):1493 (abstr)

10 Breitman T, Keene B, Hemmi H: Retinoic acid-induced differentiation of fresh human leukaemia cells and the human myelomonocytic leukaemia cell lines, HL-60, U-937, and THP-1. Cancer Surveys 1983 (2):261-291

11 Bell B, Findley H, Krischer J et al: Phase II study of 13-cis retinoic acid in pediatric patients with acute nonlymphocytic leukemia - a Pediatric Oncology Group study. J Immunotherapy 1991 (10):77-83

12 Lie S, Wathne K, Petersen L et al: High-dose retinol in children with acute myelogenous leukemia in remission. Eur J Haematol 1988 (40):460-465

13 Kramer Z, Boros L, Wiernik P et al: 13-cis retinoic acid in the treatment of elderly patients with acute myeloid leukemia. Cancer 1991 (67):1484-1486

14 Hoffman S and Robinson W: Use of differentiation-inducing agents in the myelodysplastic syndrome and acute non-lymphocytic leukemia. Am J Hematol 1988 (28):124-127

15 Hellstrom E, Rober K, Gahrton G et al: Therapeutic effects of low-dose cytosine arabinoside, alpha-interferon, 1a-hydroxyvitamin D3 and retinoic acid in acute leukemia and myeloblastic syndromes. Eur J Haematol 1988 (40):449-459

16 Hassan H and Rees J: Retinoic acid alone and in combination with cytosine arabinoside induces differentiation of human myelomonocytic and monoblastic leukemic cells. Hematological Oncology 1988 (6):39-45

17 Chomienne C, Balitrand N, Degos L et al: 1-b-d-arabinofuranosyl cytosine and all-trans retinoic acid in combination accelerates and increases monocyte differentiation of myeloid leukemic cells. Leukemia Res 1988 (10):631-636

18 Venditti A, Stasi R, Coppetelli U et al: All trans retinoic acid: effective therapy even for ANLL other than APL? Evaluation of association with low dose cytosine arabinoside. Blood 1993 (82 suppl):2186 (abstr)

19 Jakubowski A, Schuster S, Gabrilove J et al: All trans retinoic acid plus granulocyte colony stimulating factor therapy in patients with acute myelogenous leukemia - a pilot study. Blood 1993 (82 suppl):2144 (abstr)

20 Altman A: Chronic leukemias of childhood. Pediatr Clin North Am 1988 (35):765-787

21 Emanuel P, Bates L, Castleberry R et al: Selective hypersensitivity to granulocyte-macrophage colony-stimulating factor by juvenile chronic myeloid leukemia hematopoietic progenitors. Blood 1991 (77): 925-929

22 Estrov Z, Grunberger T, Chan H et al: Juvenile chronic myelogenous leukemia: Characterization of the disease using cell cultures. Blood 1986 (67): 1382-1387

23 Gualtieri R, Emanuel P, Zuckerman K et al: Granulocyte-macrophage colony-stimulating factor is an endogenous regulator of cell proliferation in juvenile chronic myelogenous leukemia. Blood 1989 (74): 2360-2367

24 Castleberry R, Emanuel P, Gualtieri R et al: Preliminary experience with 13-cis retinoic acid (cRA) in the treatment of juvenile chronic myelogenous leukemia (JCML). Blood 1991 (78):170a (abstr)

25 Sidell N, Taga T, Hirano T et al: Retinoic acid-induced growth inhibition of a human myeloma cell line via down-regulation of IL-6 receptors. J Immunol 1991 (146):3809-3814

26 Kawano M, Hirano T, Matsuda T et al: Autocrine generation and requirement of BSF-2/IL-6 for human multiple myelomas. Nature 1988 (332):83-85

27 Vesole D, Kornbluth J, Jagannath S et al: Biological response modifiers in refractory multiple myeloma: Lack of clinical efficacy of recombinant human interleukin and all-trans retinoic acid. Blood 1993 (82 suppl 1):1037 (abstr)

28 Kuzel T, Roenigk H, Rosen S: Mycosis fungoides and the Sezary syndrome: A review of pathogenesis, diagnosis, and therapy. J Clin Oncol 1991 (9):1298-1313

29 Kessler J, Levine N, Meyskens F et al: Treatment of cutaneous T-cell lymphoma (mycosis fungoides) with 13-cis retinoic acid. Lancet 1983 (1):1345-1347

30 Kessler J, Jones S, Levine N et al: Isotretinoin and cutaneous helper T-cell lymphoma (mycosis fungoides). Arch Dermatol 1987 (123):201-204

31 Molin L, Thomsen K, Volden G et al: 13-cis retinoic acid in mycosis fungoides. In: Saurat JH (ed) Retinoids: New Trends in Research and Therapy. Karger, Basel 1985 pp 341-344

32 Zachariae H and Thestrup-Pederson H: Interferon alpha and etretinate combination treatment of cutaneous T-cell lymphoma. J Invest Dermatol 1990 (95 suppl):206S-208S

33 Hoting E and Meissner K: Arotinoid-ethylester, effectiveness in refractory cutaneous T-cell lymphoma. Cancer 1988 (62):1044-1048

34 Mahrle and Thiele B: Retinoids in cutaneous T cell lymphomas. Dermatologica 1987 (175 suppl 1):145-150

35 Kuzel T, Roenigk H, Samuelson E, Rosen S: The treatment of mycosis fungoides with all-trans retinoic acid. Blood1993 (82 suppl):570a (abstr)

Retinoids in the Prevention and Therapy of Solid Tumours

Ugo Pastorino [1], David R. Parkinson [2] and Fausto Chiesa [3]

1 Department of Thoracic Surgery, Istituto Nazionale Tumori, Via Venezian 1, 20133 Milan, Italy
2 Investigational Drug Branch, Division of Cancer Treatment, National Cancer Institute, Bethesda, MD 20892, U.S.A.
3 Department of Otolaryngology, Istituto Nazionale Tumori, Via Venezian 1, 20133 Milan, Italy

The biology and results of preclinical studies with retinoids suggest that they may be useful in both the prevention and treatment of malignancy. Cancer prevention research is rapidly developing, and retinoids have played a crucial role in the first successful attempts to antagonise the process of carcinogenesis. Experimentally, there is now little doubt that chemoprevention with retinoids is feasible, but the nature and extent of the biological effects of retinoids on human carcinogenesis still demand extensive investigation.

In humans, the model of multistep carcinogenesis implies that invasive cancer is the ultimate product of a sequence of critical events, many (if not all) of which could theoretically be prevented (Fig. 1). The broad spectrum of possible preventive measures includes the inhibition of early induction phases, such as metabolic activation or DNA binding, but consists mainly of a permanent suppression of the long promotion phase. In fact the epidemiological phenomenon of latency opens a large window (up to 20 years) for prevention purposes. Biological understanding of the carcinogenic process in the various fields (i.e., upper aerodigestive, colorectal, mammary, urothelial) has significantly improved as a consequence of chemoprevention research.

In some ways, chemoprevention represents an evolution of traditional systemic chemotherapy. The cytolytic approach to the disease is replaced by approaches which involve induction of differentiation, cytostasis and apoptosis, but the ultimate goal remains similar: to provide an effective medical treatment for those solid tumours which are highly chemoresistant. As for the screening of new anticancer drugs, specific experimental models have had to be set up for retinoids and other chemopreventive agents, representing at best the various risk populations, target tissues/organs, and mechanisms of environmental carcinogenesis.

The clinical field of chemoprevention is relatively recent, and the nature of the trials is that they take considerable time to complete. As a result, only a few major chemoprevention trials have been concluded, while most of them are

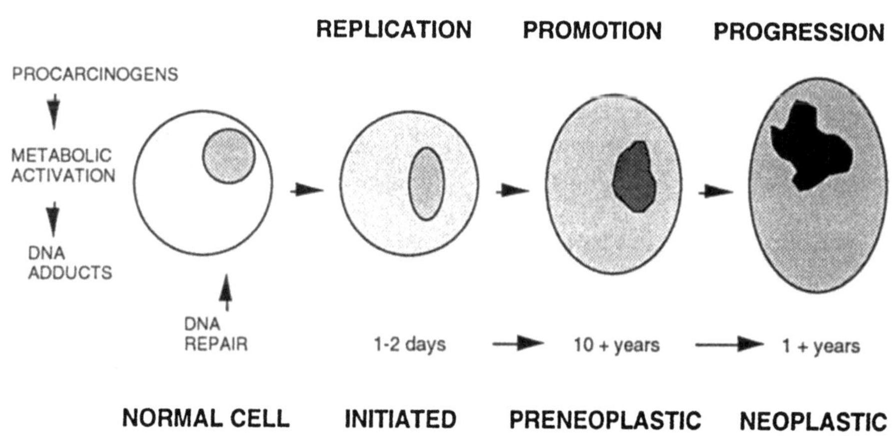

Fig. 1. Hypothetical phases of multistep carcinogenic process

still ongoing. These trials are expected to provide substantial information regarding crucial aspects of chemoprevention: optimal selection of target populations, choice of preventive agent(s), dose and duration of treatment, and definition of specific endpoints. For the time being, cancer chemoprevention has to be considered an experimental procedure, to be performed under strict clinical control and proper methodology of evaluation.
The use of retinoids in treatment of malignancies has been relatively limited until recently. However, the success of therapy of acute promyelocytic leukaemia with all-*trans* retinoic acid has stimulated interest in retinoid therapy of solid tumours as well.

Methodological Aspects of Chemoprevention

Selection of High-Risk Individuals

Three different levels of chemoprevention intervention can be defined: primary chemoprevention, treatment of precancerous lesions, and secondary chemoprevention. Based on epidemiologic and experimental data, primary chemoprevention trials in healthy individuals aim at interfering with the early phases of carcinogenesis by counteracting a hypothetical deficiency of putative protective agents. With respect to lung cancer, for example, the target population is represented by otherwise healthy individuals at high risk of developing lung cancer because of previous heavy exposure to smoking, asbestos, or other carcinogens. The nature of these primary chemoprevention studies is that they have to recruit many thousands of people to reach an adequate number of events. Other limiting factors are represented by the long period of observation (5-10 years), the low doses of preventive agents, and the double-blind setting. Since a major concern involves minimising the risk of harmful effects to the population under treatment, the long-term tolerability of the intervention plan is of critical importance.
The second level of chemoprevention intervention involves subjects affected by precancerous or preinvasive lesions such as oral leukoplakia, cervical dysplasia, colorectal adenoma, bronchial metaplasia, or actinic keratosis. The aim of the treatment in this case is regression of preneoplastic disease and prevention of progression to invasive cancer. Such studies are usually conducted with double-blind randomisation and involve a relatively limited number of patients.
Secondary chemoprevention is aimed at preventing the occurrence of new primary tumours in patients cured of a prior cancer and known to be at higher risk for a second cancer. Multiple primary tumours may occur in the upper aerodigestive tract due to widespread exposure of the epithelium to common aetiological factors such as tobacco smoking and other environmental carcinogens [1,2]. Dietary habits may also play a role in this process as a modifier of the individual risk of cancer. This clinical evidence finds its biological rationale in the concept of "field cancerisation", suggesting that repeated exposure of the entire epithelial surface to carcinogenic insults may result in the occurrence of multiple, independent premalignant or malignant foci [3].
In patients cured of a cancer of the oral cavity, larynx, lung, oesophagus or bladder, the lifetime incidence of second primary tumours in all sites is 10-35% (or 2 to 6% per year), depending on the site, histological type and stage of the index tumour; in patients with a good initial prognosis these second tumours may represent a significant cause of failure [4-6]. Compared to healthy subjects, patients cured of a prior cancer are more highly motivated to accept the extra burden of a chemoprevention treatment strategy, as an extension of long-term follow-up planned for their index tumour (Table 1). They are more likely to tolerate the side-effects associated with chemopreventive therapy, and higher doses can therefore be given in order to achieve a potential adjuvant effect against primary cancer relapse.
For all the above reasons, patients treated curatively for a prior cancer of the upper aerodigestive tract are an ideal population in which to test the efficacy of chemopreventive agents (retinoids, vitamins and antioxidants), either alone or in combination with other adjuvant treatments [7,8]. Of particular interest to chemoprevention purposes is the fact that significant genetic changes may be detectable with various degrees of severity in bronchial dysplasia as well as in pathologically normal mucosa [9,10]. For example, patients with mul-

Table 1. Comparison between studies on healthy populations (primary chemoprevention) and studies on patients with prior cancer (secondary chemoprevention)

	Chemoprevention Primary	Secondary
Selection criteria	Prior exposure	Prior cancer
Phase of carcinogenesis	Initial (induction)	Late (promotion)
Risk of cancer	Limited (< 0.5% / year)	High (1-3% / year)
Sample size	Thousands	Hundreds
Pharmacological dose	Minimal (effective)	Maximal (tolerable)
Duration of intervention	Years	Months
Control group	Double-blind or placebo	Placebo or no treatment
Side-effects	Absent	Significant
Follow-up	Long interval	Short interval
Biological monitoring	Difficult	Easy
Costs (additional)	High	Limited

tiple tumours of the upper aerodigestive tract, either synchronous or metachronous, show a much higher frequency of genetic changes compared to those with single or multiple tumours at other sites [11].

These data indicate that specific genetic abnormalities may be detectable in the various stages of lung tumorigenesis, in a sequence of events ranging all the way from normal epithelium to bronchial metaplasia and dysplasia, carcinoma *in situ*, early stage invasive cancer, and ultimately ending in locally advanced and metastatic lung cancer.

In practical terms, it is conceivable that a panel of specific markers, including chromosome deletions (3p, 7p, 17), P53 staining, epithelial growth factor receptor (EGFR) and the oncogene HER2/neu, will be used to select future candidates for chemoprevention programmes. In fact, with the development of immunostaining techniques for fresh and paraffin-embedded tissues, fluorescence *in situ* hybridisation (FISH) and polymerase chain reaction (PCR) for selective chromosome testing, even small samples collected through bronchoscopic biopsies, brushing or sputum cytology, will become suitable for the screening of high-risk individuals appropriate for chemoprevention trials.

Endpoints

The final goal of chemoprevention is clearly the improvement of survival. However, given the enormous costs and length of time required to demonstrate a survival benefit in clinical trials, it has become mandatory to identify a few intermediate endpoints to help answer some of the various open questions in this field, such as selection of the most active agents, the dose and duration of treatment. As shown by recent experiences, even a biologically important success such as the significant reduction of the incidence of second primary tumours may not translate into improved survival, due to comorbidity and/or salvage treatment of second primaries in the control group. At the clinical level, therefore, it is important to define the overall benefit of intervention, namely an improvement in survival, having adjusted for competing risks of death, in order to balance this benefit against the toxicities and other costs of therapy.

A problem with the interpretation of the results of chemoprevention trials has been that in secondary chemoprevention, a differential diagnosis of second primary tumours from recurrences of prior disease can be difficult, and traditional criteria based on the anatomical site (distance from prior cancer), histological type (same vs. different), and temporal sequence (time elapsed from prior cancer) may be elusive. Recent findings suggest that the study of biological markers (3p deletion, LOH 3p, P53 or K-ras mutations) may improve the differential diagnosis of multiple primary tumours occurring in the same area [12].

As noted, the identification of appropriate in-

Table 2. Intermediate biomarkers in cancer chemoprevention

Genetic markers	Micronuclei Ploidy and DNA content Chromosome deletions/translocations Oncogene activation
Differentiation markers	Squamous markers (keratins, involucrin) Blood group antigens
Proliferation markers	Proliferating Cell Nuclear Antigen (PCNA) Thymidine Labeling Index Retinoic Acid Receptors (RARs) Epidermal Growth Factor Receptor (EGFR) Transforming Growth Factor-ß (TGF-ß)

termediate endpoints is another crucial aspect of cancer chemoprevention research. Appropriate biological intermediate endpoints are essential to monitor the biological effects of preventive strategies before the actual occurrence of invasive cancer [13]. In order to justify systematic application, such intermediate endpoints need to be: a) specific for the process of carcinogenesis under study; b) quantitatively or qualitatively correlated with the degree of progression; c) easily measurable on small specimens, which can be obtained in a tolerable manner from the subject at repeated intervals; d) potentially modulated by the selected preventive agent. Potential intermediate biomarkers which are under investigation may be grouped into 3 categories: genetic markers, differentiation markers and proliferation markers (Table 2).

Similarly, many of the ongoing trials of retinoids in the treatment of established solid tumours include ancillary studies to help define the biological effects of the retinoids on the tumour cells. Following is a discussion of the current status of clinical investigations of the use of retinoids in the prevention and treatment of solid tumours.

Skin Cancer

Chemoprevention of Skin Cancer with Retinoids

The efficacy of retinoids in the treatment of non-malignant dermatological diseases and the biological rationales suggesting their ability to block the malignant process, have made these substances important therapeutic agents in the therapy of cutaneous precancerous lesions.

In actinic keratosis, topical administration of 13-*cis* RA led to complete remission (CR) in 40% to 50% of patients, with overall objective response (OR) rates in the 75-95% range [8]. Similar results were obtained in a pilot study with oral etretinate at a daily dose of 1 mg/kg (CR 75%, OR 95%), and subsequently confirmed by double-blind randomised trials using etretinate at the dose of 75 mg/day for 2 months [14] or 1 mg/kg for 4 months [15].

A small study involving patients with xeroderma pigmentosum demonstrated that 2-year treatment with high-dose 13-*cis* RA (2 mg/kg/day) was able to induce nearly total suppression of the occurrence of basal cell carcinomas of the skin [16]. Unfortunately, the basal cancer incidence rates returned to the initial level soon after 13-*cis* RA treatment was interrupted. Nonetheless, the positive results obtained in such an aggressive premalignant disease have given considerable support to the initiation of large-scale preventive trials in patients with a history of prior skin cancer. One of these studies, involving 981 patients previously treated for two or more basal cell carcinomas of the skin, has been concluded recently [17]. In this trial, oral administration of 13-*cis* RA at a daily dose of 10 mg for 36 months failed to reduce the occurrence of basal cell carcinoma at new sites when compared with placebo. Criticism regarding this trial was related to the drug schedule, since it involved a daily dose of 13-*cis* RA far below the usual range. Quite surprisingly with such a low dose, the authors still reported a significant ex-

Table 3. Chemoprevention trials on skin cancer* using retinoids as preventive agent

Investigator	Population	Agent	Dose	No. subjects	Endpoint
Precancerous diseases					
Moon (USA)	Actinic keratosis	Retinol	25,000 IU/day	2800	Basal cell carcinoma, squamous carcinoma
Secondary chemoprevention					
Clark (USA)	Prior skin cancer	Selenium Retinol Vitamin E	400 μg/day 50,000 IU/day 0.1 mg/day	400	Basal cell carcinoma, squamous carcinoma
Moon (USA)	Prior (4+) skin cancer	Retinol 13-*cis* RA	25,000 IU/day 5-10 mg/day	500	Basal cell carcinoma, squamous carcinoma
Nava (Italy)	Prior skin cancer	4-HPR	200 mg/day	900	Basal cell carcinoma, squamous carcinoma

* excluding malignant melanoma

cess of toxicity (elevated serum triglycerides, hyperostotic axial skeletal changes, and mucocutaneous reactions) in the treated group.

As illustrated in Table 3, several studies are currently ongoing both in patients with precancerous lesions and in high-risk individuals, involving various populations and intervention programmes. The study currently activated in Milan is testing the effectiveness of the oral administration of 4-HPR (200 mg/day for 1 year) in decreasing recurrences and preventing new tumours after radical excision of basal cell carcinoma. The trial is restricted to patients with tumours located in the head and neck area, where surgical management of recurrences may be more difficult and mutilating. By March 1994, a total of 730 patients were randomised (363 in the 4-HPR group and 367 in the control group) [18].

Treatment of Squamous Cell Carcinoma of the Skin with Retinoids

Based on preclinical data suggesting that the combination of retinoids and interferon alpha may have advantages [19], Lippman et al. initiated a clinical trial in patients with advanced squamous cell carcinoma of the skin [20]. Patients were eligible for treatment if standard local therapy with surgery and/or radiotherapy had failed, if such therapy was not technically feasible or acceptable due to tumour size, location, or involvement of adjacent structures, or if the cancer had metastasized to regional or distant sites. Of the 32 patients entered into the study, 28 were eligible for response. In general, patients had been heavily pretreated, either with multiple resections including radical neck dissection, or with radiotherapy, or with chemotherapy (6 patients). Patients were treated with recombinant interferon alpha-2a (IFN-α, Roferon-A, Hoffmann-La Roche, Basle) administered at 3 million units daily, and 13-*cis* retinoic acid (13-*cis* RA, Accutane, Hoffman-La Roche) administered orally at 1 mg/kg daily. Toxicities of this combination reflected the individual toxicities of the component agents. Grade 3 fatigue was observed in 12 patients, and grade 2 or greater flu-like syndrome in 12 patients. The overall response rate was 68% in the evaluable patients; 7 of the 19 responding patients achieved a complete response. Patients with less advanced disease had a greater likelihood of response: 13 of 14 patients with locally advanced disease, 4 of 6 patients with regional disease, and 2 of 8 patients with metastatic disease responded. While it is not possible from these small numbers to determine whether synergistic activity has taken place, the nonetheless promising combination therapy results are consistent with the cell culture data and have stimulated great interest in the combined use of these two agents [21].

In a more recent experience with the same regimen in patients with advanced SCC at different sites, Toma et al. [22] also observed activity in SCC of the skin, with 3 responses in 6 evaluable patients. These investigators also obtained responses in SCC at other sites including head and neck, lung, vulva, and, of particular interest, complete responses in 1 patient with carcinoma of the penis and 2 patients with SCC of the oesophagus.

Treatment of Basal Cell Carcinoma with Retinoids

Both 13-*cis* RA and RA have been used topically in the therapy of cutaneous basal cell carcinoma. Several studies have documented that most patients exhibit partial or complete regression of their lesions [23]. Systemic 13-*cis* RA has shown efficacy, although at doses associated with both acute and chronic toxicity. In a study published by Peck et al. [24] mean daily 13-*cis* RA doses of 3.1 mg/kg administered to 12 patients were associated with a greater than one third response rate, and histologically confirmed complete regression occurred in approximatey 10% of tumours. Oral etretinate was also reported to have activity in patients with multiple basal cell carcinomas [25]. In this study, decreased rates of new tumour formation were noted in patients with conditions predisposing to the development of basal cell carcinomas (arsenical insecticide exposure or nevoid basal cell carcinoma syndrome) who were treated with 13-*cis* RA, with higher rates of tumour development again observed either at lower doses or at discontinuation of therapy.

Malignant Melanoma

In vitro, retinoids are capable of inhibiting the growth of murine and human melanoma cells, and retinoids can inhibit the development of melanoma metastases in athymic mice [26]. However, a single melanoma cell line responded differentially to different retinoids, and different melanoma cell lines showed very different patterns of response to RA exposure, indicating heterogeneity in the biological response [27]. One study suggested that part of this variation in response may be related to differences in expression of retinoic acid receptors, with lines expressing RAR beta more sensitive to RA than those which did not [28].

Treatment of Malignant Melanoma with Retinoids

Consistent with the preclinical data, some limited antitumour activity has been observed with retinoids in therapy of established melanoma. Topical application of RA to subcutaneous metastatic melanoma lesions resulted in transient local regression of some tumours [29]. Partial tumour responses in 3 of 20 patients with advanced metastatic malignant melanoma were noted using systemic 13-*cis* RA at 2-3 mg/kg [8]. Retinol (200,000 IU/m^2/d) resulted in an objective response in 1 of 15 patients treated [30]. Fenretinide (4-HPR) was inactive in a phase II trial in patients with advanced melanoma [31].

There is limited clinical experience with retinoids in the adjuvant therapy of melanoma. A randomised phase III trial of oral retinol (100,000 IU/d for 18 months) was conducted in patients with stage I melanoma; initial evaluation suggested no benefit to either relapse-free or overall survival [32].

Based on the preclinical data and the initial clinical experience in some SCCs discussed earlier, a phase II trial of the combination of interferon alpha and 13-*cis* RA was performed in 11 patients with metastatic melanoma. All patients had progressed after combination chemotherapy. In 10 evaluable patients the therapy was well tolerated, but no objective responses were achieved [33].

Head and Neck Cancer

Chemoprevention of Head and Neck Cancer with Retinoids

Great interest and high expectations for the successful chemoprevention of premalignant lesions in the upper aerodigestive tract have been generated by the results of the initial clinical studies in oral leukoplakia. In the last decade, oral leukoplakia has represented the most reliable clinical model in which to test the direct, short-term efficacy of chemopreventive agents. The path-finding clinical trials conducted at the M.D. Anderson Cancer Center are of fundamental importance because of the strict methodological criteria applied: randomised, double-blind setting and detailed pathological assessment of both pre-randomisation status and response to treatment. The first study demonstrated that treatment with 13-*cis* retinoic acid (1-2 mg/kg daily for 3 months) could result in major regression of leukoplakia in 67% of patients (vs. 10% for placebo); however, relapse occurred in most cases soon after cessation of treatment [34]. A further study of isotretinoin was then designed to overcome the dual problem of significant toxicity and rapid recurrence. In this trial, patients received an induction treatment with high-dose isotretinoin (1.5 mg/kg per day) for a 3-month induction period and were then randomised to a 9-month maintenance therapy with either low-dose isotretinoin (0.5 mg/kg/d) or beta-carotene (30 mg/d). This study showed that low-dose isotretinoin was significantly more effective than beta-carotene in maintaining clinical/histological remission (relapse rate of 6% vs. 58%), thus demonstrating that low-dose isotretinoin was an effective and well-tolerated maintenance therapy for oral premalignancy [35].

Other studies of oral leukoplakia are ongoing (Table 4). One of these trials is accruing patients with prior leukoplakia which has been surgically resected by laser. Patients are randomised to treatment with 4-HPR (200 mg/day for 1 year) with the aim of preventing new leukoplakia lesions, recurrence of excised leukoplakia, and development of frank oral cancer. The preliminary results showed a significant reduction in the incidence of new leukoplakia lesions [36], and a recent update has confirmed the above results. During the year of intervention 14 patients had recurrences (9 in the control group and 5 in the 4-HPR group) and 10 showed development of new leukoplasia lesions (9 in the control group and 1 in the 4-HPR group). The overall risk of recurrence and new lesions in the patients who completed the intervention was 6% in the 4-HPR group and 30% in the control group ($p = 0.009$).

The pioneering study of chemoprevention of second primary tumours was conducted in patients with a history of treated squamous cell carcinoma of the head and neck. All patients had been previously treated with surgery, radiotherapy, or both. Following stratification by tumour site (oral cavity, oropharynx, hypopharynx, or larynx) and prior treatment (sur-

Table 4. Chemoprevention trials on head and neck cancer using retinoids as preventive agent

Investigator	Population	Agent	Dose	No. subjects	Endpoint
Precancerous diseases					
Lippman (USA)	Oral leukoplakia	Beta-carotene + retinol versus 13-*cis* RA	30 mg/day 25,000 IU/day 0.5-0.25 mg/kg/day	600	Regression, oral cancer, micronuclei
Chiesa (Milano)	Oral leukoplakia resected	4-HPR	200 mg/day	300	Recurrence, new lesions, oral cancer
Zaridze (Uzbekistan)	Oral leukoplakia, chronic oesophagitis	Retinol Beta-carotene Riboflavin	30 mg/week 280 mg/week 200 mg/week	800	Oral cancer, micronuclei
Secondary chemoprevention					
Intergroup (USA)	Head & neck cancer stage I	13-*cis* RA	30 mg/day	1000	Second primary tumours
EUROSCAN (Europe)	Squamous cancer larynx and oral cavity stage I-III	Retinyl palmitate N-acetylcysteine	300,000 IU 600 mg/day	2500*	Second primary tumours, survival

* including lung cancer patients

gery, radiation, combined), patients were randomised to receive either 13-*cis* RA (50 to 100 mg/m^2/day) or placebo for 12 months. The study was closed after enrollment of a total of 103 cases. The endpoints of this study included both recurrence of primary disease and development of second primary tumours. After a median follow-up of 32 months, the first analysis showed that retinoid treatment significantly reduced the incidence of second primary tumours [37]. Only 2 patients (4%) in the retinoid arm developed second primary tumours versus 12 patients (24%) in the placebo arm ($p = 0.005$). Most second primaries (13/14, 93%) occurred in the head and neck, oesophagus, or lung. Treatment-related toxicity was significant, and 33% (16/49) of the isotretinoin patients could not complete the 12-month schedule. A recently updated analysis, with a 54-month median follow-up, confirmed the reduction in second primary tumours: 7 patients (14%) in the retinoid arm versus 16 patients (31%) in the placebo arm, but the difference was less striking ($p = 0.04$) [38].

A concurrent study was conducted from 1985 to 1991 by a French cooperative group (GETEC): 323 patients with a squamous cancer of the oral cavity and oropharynx (T1-2 N0-1) which had been treated for cure were randomised to receive a synthetic retinoid (etretinate, oral 25 mg daily, 24 months) or placebo. The endpoint of this study was total survival. The analysis of this trial has been performed recently and formal publication is forthcoming. Preliminary reports are negative in terms of efficacy: both survival and occurrence of second primary tumours are similar in the two arms [39].

In an attempt to confirm the positive results of the first M.D. Anderson study with 13-*cis* RA, two large scale trials are under way (Table 4). One has been developed by the Radiation Therapy Oncology Group (RTOG), in cooperation with the Community Clinical Oncology Program (CCOP - M.D. Anderson). Patients with prior head and neck cancer (stage I and II) are being treated with low-dose 13-*cis* RA (30 mg/day) or placebo, for 3 years. The other study, denominated EUROSCAN, is ongoing in Europe on patients treated for cancer of the lung, larynx and oral cavity. Details are provided in the lung cancer section of this chapter.

Treatment of Head and Neck Cancer with Retinoids

Retinoids have been demonstrated to have antiproliferative and differentiative effects on SCC cell lines and multicellular SCC tumour spheroids from patients with head and neck carcinoma [40]. Phase II studies conducted on the basis of the preclinical rationale have indicated some activity of these agents in patients with advanced disease; partial responses of short duration were induced in patients with advanced head and neck cancer with 13-*cis* RA (3 mg/kg/d) in 3 of 19 patients in one study [41,42]. In a second, randomised phase II study of patients with locally advanced or metastatic head and neck SCC, the observation was again made that 3 of 19 responded to 13-*cis* RA at the same dose as that used in the previous study, with one patient achieving a complete response [43].

The use of retinoids in combination therapy in clinical trials involving patients with head and neck cancer has been studied to some extent. Vitamin A and 5-fluorouracil were administered together with external-beam irradiation (FAR therapy) in a Japanese study [44]; the authors suggest that this therapy was superior to radiation alone based on the comparison of survival results between 250 patients treated primarily with this combination and a site-specific historical control group. Both a British study using vitamin A administered together with combination chemotherapy including doxorubicin, bleomycin, 5-fluorouracil, and methotrexate [45], and a second study using beta-carotene together with chemotherapy and radiation therapy suggested that concomitant use of retinoids may decrease the mucositis associated with these therapies [46].

Based on the observations described above which suggest some single-agent activity for retinoids in SCC of the head and neck, together with findings indicating that interferon-alpha has limited activity in the same setting and the demonstrated efficacy of the combination of IFN-alpha and 13-*cis* RA in SCC of the skin or cervix, a phase II study of the same combination was performed in 21 evaluable patients with recurrent squamous cell carcinoma of the head and neck [47]. All patients had received previous treatment with either chemotherapy or radiation therapy. Only a single partial response was noted in this group. Five of the patients developed grade 3 toxicities, including skin toxicities, fatigue, headache, and anorexia with weight loss. The median survival of 25.5 weeks was similar to that expected in patients with recurrent head and neck carcinoma treated with cytotoxic chemotherapy. The investigators concluded that this regimen was inactive in recurrent squamous cell carcinoma of the head and neck. These results suggest that the observation of retinoid therapeutic activity in SCC arising in skin or cervix cannot be immediately generalised to all SCC. Additionally, this head and neck cancer patient population did not tolerate the combination therapy well. The role of pretreatment with radiation and/or chemotherapy in decreasing the likelihood of response to this form of therapy, as in the case of cervical carcinoma discussed below, remains unclear.

Consistent with the above observations suggesting little activity of currently studied retinoids in head and neck SCC, were the findings of the above-mentioned chemoprevention study where 13-*cis* RA therapy (50-100 mg/m^2/d) significantly decreased the incidence of second epithelial tumours but did not affect the incidence of recurrence of metastases from the primary tumour [37].

Lung Cancer

Lung Cancer Chemoprevention

Table 5 summarises the ongoing trials of primary lung cancer chemoprevention. The majority of these studies were designed and launched in the early 1980s, funded by the Chemoprevention Branch of the National Cancer Institute [48]. In these studies, low-dose retinol (25,000 IU/day) is administered in combination with beta-carotene, vitamin E, or selenium. The main endpoint of these trials is the prevention of lung cancer in a population of high-risk individuals.

Interest in the use of retinoids for the treatment of precancerous lesions of bronchial epithelium was generated by the data on oral premalignancy discussed earlier, and 2 randomised trials were conducted on heavy-smoker volunteers with bronchial metaplasia. The first study tested the efficacy of etretinate on sputum cytology of heavy smokers. After 6 months of treatment, the degree of atypia measured in the sputum of etretinate-treated subjects was similar to that observed in the placebo group [49]. In the second trial, conducted at the M.D. Anderson Cancer Center, 87 chronic smokers with bronchial dysplasia and/or metaplasia greater than 15% as assessed by multiple bronchoscopic biopsies (6 sites), were randomised to either 13-*cis* retinoic acid (1 mg/kg/day) or placebo. Bronchoscopic re-evaluation at 6 months, available for 67 subjects, showed a similar decrease in the frequency of squamous metaplasia in both arms (55% vs. 59%), with the reduction being more pronounced in those who had stopped smoking [50]. This study, although negative in terms of treatment efficacy, has provided essential information on the natural history of bronchial metaplasia, and underlines the importance of conducting properly controlled trials. A third study is currently testing the efficacy of 4-HPR in a similar setting.

The first randomised clinical trial of secondary lung cancer chemoprevention was started in 1985 at the Instituto Nazionale Tumori of Milan. Patients with pathological stage 1 (T1-T2, N0, M0) non-small cell lung carcinoma following complete surgical resection were selected for this study. Patients were randomly assigned to either vitamin A treatment (oral 300,000 I.U. daily, 12 to 24 months) or to control observation, stratified according to the centre, cell type (squamous versus non-squamous) and previous cancer at another site (absent versus cured). The endpoints of this study were: relapse of prior cancer, occurrence of new primary cancers, and survival. The accrual was closed in 1989 with 307 evaluable patients, and the results of multivariate analysis, based on a median follow-up of 46 months, have been published recently [51]. In summary, 56 (37%) patients in the treated arm developed either recurrence or new primary tumours, against 75 (48%) in the control arm. Eighteen patients (12%) in the treated group developed a second primary tumour, and 29 patients in the control group developed 33 (21%) second primary tumours. The estimated proportion of patients disease-free at 5 years was 64% vs. 51% in favour of the treatment arm; the difference was significant when adjusted for primary tumour classification ($p = 0.038$). A statistically significant difference was also observed in the

Table 5. Chemoprevention trials on lung cancer using retinoids as preventive agent

Investigator	Population	Agent	Dose	No. subjects	Endpoint
Primary chemoprevention					
Goodman (Seattle)	Smokers 50-69 years	Beta-carotene Retinol	30 mg/day 25,000 IU/day	13,000	Lung cancer
Omenn (Seattle)	Asbestos workers, smokers, 45-69 yrs	Beta-carotene Retinol	30 mg/day 25,000 IU/day	4,000	Lung cancer
Mclarty (Tyler)	Asbestos workers	Beta-carotene Retinol	50 mg/day 25,000 IU/day	600	Lung cancer
Xuan (China)	Tin miners	Retinol Beta-carotene Vitamin E Selenium	25,000 IU/day 50 mg/ day 800 IU/day 400 ug/day	7000	Lung cancer
Precancerous diseases					
Brenner (USA)	Bronchial metaplasia index > 15%	4-HPR	200 mg/day	100	Metaplasia, dysplasia, biological markers
Secondary chemoprevention					
Intergroup (USA)	NSCLC stage I	13-*cis* RA	30 mg/day	600	Second primary tumours
EUROSCAN (Europe)	NSCLC stage I-III	Retinyl palmitate N-acetylcysteine	300,000 IU 600 mg/day	2500*	Second primary tumours, survival

NSCLC, non-small cell lung cancer
* including head and neck cancer patients

time to new primaries in the field of prevention, i.e., tobacco-related tumours (p = 0.045, log rank test), and in the estimated proportion of patients free of new primaries in the field (89% vs. 80%, p = 0.045). In terms of toxicity and side-effects, high-dose vitamin A proved to be a relatively safe treatment, well tolerated for a period of 1 to 2 years, with an overall compliance rate of nearly 80%.

As a follow-up to this trial, a new European cooperative study ("EUROSCAN") was set up in 1988 as a joint venture of the E.O.R.T.C. Lung Cancer and Head and Neck Cancer Cooperative Groups [52], to test the combination of 2 agents with different preventive properties: retinol palmitate and n-acetyl-cysteine (NAC). The goal of the EUROSCAN study was the prevention of second primary tumours in patients treated for upper aero-digestive tract cancer. Eligible patients were those previously treated for squamous cancer of the larynx (Tis, T1-2-3, N0-1), squamous cancer of the oral cavity (T1-2, N0-1), or non-small cell lung cancer (pT1-2, N0-1 and T3 NO). Four treatment arms were planned in a 2 x 2 factorial design, to increase efficiency and power: a) retinol palmitate and NAC; b) retinol palmitate; c) NAC; d) no treatment. Randomisation takes place after surgery and/or completion of radiotherapy. Retinol palmitate is administered at a daily oral dose of 300,000 IU for the first 12 months, followed by 150,000 IU for 12 additional months. NAC is administered at a daily dose of 600 mg for 2 years. Minimal follow-up includes physical examination 3-monthly and chest X-ray 6-monthly. The endpoints of this study are: relapse of prior cancer, occurrence of new primary cancers, and survival. By April 1993, all the initially planned 2000 patients had entered the trial, but it was decided to prolong the accrual up to a total of 2500 patients.

The interest generated by the above trials has led to a new independent study promoted by the U.S. Intergroup in 1992 on resected stage I non-small cell lung carcinoma. This trial is expected to enter over 600 patients, randomised to either oral 13-*cis* RA (30 mg/day) or placebo [53].

Treatment of Non-Small Cell Lung Cancer (NSCLC) with Retinoids

RA inhibited clonal proliferation in 7 of 9 non-small cell lung cancer cell lines, which suggests that this tumour type might be responsive [54]. However, clinical studies of 13-*cis* RA, retinyl palmitate, or retinol in patients with advanced NSCLC have been associated with objective tumour responses in less than 10% of treated patients [30,41,55-56]. In a more recent study, Rinaldi et al. reported on the results of a phase II trial of the combination of 13-*cis* RA and interferon alpha-2a in advanced SCC of the lung; 17 of the 21 patients enrolled were evaluable for response, 4 with locally advanced and 13 with metastatic disease. The therapy was not well tolerated by this group of patients, with almost half of the patients discontinuing therapy due to side-effects. A single partial response was achieved in this group of patients, suggesting that, similar to the situation with SCC of the head and neck, this tumour will not show the same sensitivity as observed with SCC of the skin.

Treatment of Small Cell Lung Cancer (SCLC) with Retinoids

In one preclinical study, small cell lung cancer cell lines showed minimal growth inhibition following exposure to RA; however, in another study which involved the use of variant SCLC cell lines, the malignant cells were sensitive to the differentiation effects of RA, as indicated by their acquisition of morphological and some biological characteristics of classic SCLC cell lines [57]. The same group studied the interaction between retinoids and cytotoxic chemotherapy on SCLC cells; while the sensitivity of SCLC cells to etoposide was increased, that to doxorubicin was decreased. There are clinical trials under way to explore the use of retinoids together with chemotherapy in the treatment of both small cell and non-small cell carcinoma, with no published results as yet.

Retinoids in the Treatment of Cervical Cancer

Lippman et al. reported on the therapeutic results of a combination of interferon-alpha 2a and 13-*cis* retinoic acid utilising the same dose and schedule as they had used in the treatment of squamous cell carcinoma of the skin [58,59]. The regimen was well tolerated in the predominantly young group of women treated in Guadalajara, Mexico. The women all had locally advanced cervical carcinoma, were HIV negative, and had not received prior therapy with either chemotherapy or radiation. The toxicities of this outpatient regimen consisted of transient flu-like syndrome, cheilitis, dry skin, hypertriglyceridaemia, fatigue and anorexia. Of the 26 patients treated, 13 (50%) achieved objective responses, among which one complete response. Overall, the response rate was 58% in patients with IIB or higher-grade disease; responses did occur, although at lower frequency, in patients with bulky disease. In the second report, with an update and extension of the analysis to a total of 32 treated patients, the same response rates were obtained, with a total of 5 pathologically confirmed complete responses. The median time to response in this study was only 1 month, with a median duration of response of 3 months. As a result of the high response rates and relatively short response duration in these previously untreated patients, subsequent clinical trials are examining the value of this regimen as neoadjuvant therapy and as a radiation sensitizer in advanced disease.

Breast Cancer

Preclinical studies support the possibility that retinoid-based therapy may find a place in the chemoprevention or treatment of breast carcinoma. Several studies have documented the inhibition of human breast cancer cell lines by retinoids [60,61]. This inhibition has been observed most often with oestrogen-dependent cell lines, and Fontana et al. have suggested a correlation between retinoid responsiveness and inhibition by retinoids of a 39 kD protein associated with oestrogen dependence [62]. Dietary supplementation with RA in rats with

nitrosourea-induced mammary tumours decreased the progression rate of the tumours without adding to the tumour regression induced by ovariectomy [63]. Of interest was the observation by Halter et al. that while *in vitro* both RA and 13-*cis* RA were effective in inhibiting the growth of a human mammary carcinoma cell line, only RA was able to prevent growth of xenotransplanted carcinoma cells in athymic mice, additional evidence for functional distinctions between these two retinoids [64].
Another retinoid of specific interest for breast cancer chemoprevention is 4-HPR (fenretinide) [65]. 4-HPR was shown to accumulate preferentially in the breast rather than the liver [66], and to inhibit chemically induced mammary carcinoma in rats [67]. Preliminary studies in Sprague-Dawley rats showed that combined treatment with 4-HPR plus tamoxifen is superior to either agent alone in blocking progression of neoplastic lesions [68].

Breast Cancer Chemoprevention

On the basis of this experimental evidence, 4-HPR has been selected for the first trial on human breast cancer chemoprevention [69]. The clinical background for this approach included the observation that patients treated for an early stage breast cancer had an excellent prognosis (about 80-90% survival), but also a definite risk of developing a contralateral breast cancer, representing an independent biological event. This incidence of contralateral breast cancer was in the order of 0.8% per year, and remained stable during the first 10 years after surgical excision of the primary breast cancer.
A large randomised clinical trial was initiated in 1987 at the Istituto Tumori of Milan in patients who had been operated on for stage I oestrogen-receptor positive (ER+) breast cancer, with the aim of reducing the incidence of contralateral breast cancer. Eligible patients were randomised to oral administration of 4-HPR (200 mg/day for 5 years) or to a control arm without treatment. A 3-day drug holiday was applied at the end of each month, in order to avoid some of the adverse effects possibly related to a prolonged decrease in plasma levels of retinol [70,71].
By the end of 1993, nearly 3,000 patients had been randomised, and accrual was closed on 30th June. Compliance and tolerability of the drug remained very good during the study. Notwithstanding the large number of patients entered, at this writing the follow-up is still too short to draw any meaningful conclusion regarding the preventive effect of 4-HPR. In fact, contralateral primaries appearing in the first 3 years of intervention are likely to be present at the time of randomisation, even though too small to be detected by physical examination and mammography. A preliminary interim analysis performed in August 1994 shows a slight benefit from 4-HPR intake only in the group of patients below 45 years of age and mainly during exposure to the agent. More than one-third of the subjects are still on intervention and further time is required to draw more solid conclusions.
As noted, the drug was well tolerated and only a small minority of patients (3%) interrupted the 4-HPR treatment for proven toxicity or related complaints. At initial analysis, fifty-three (34 in the 4-HPR group and 19 in the control group) subjects had dropped out due to intercurrent events (not related to the disease) and 111 of the 4-HPR group for refusal. A total of 272 patients (129 in the 4-HPR group and 143 in the control group) had dropped out on the basis of tumour relapse [72]. No acute toxicity was observed when the retinoid was administered orally at a daily dose of 200 mg. The dermatological tolerability was very good, and no liver function abnormalities were observed. The 3-day drug holiday at the end of each month has apparently proven effective in preventing the impaired dark adaptation due to a significant drop in plasma retinol levels [70-72].
Independent of the results which will be observed in this study, the data already available on the efficacy of tamoxifen in an adjuvant setting [73,74], as well as the apparent synergy between tamoxifen and 4-HPR observed in experimental carcinogenesis, suggest that a clinical evaluation of the combination of 4-HPR and tamoxifen is worthwhile studying in the chemoprevention setting. Such trials are currently under design in the United States, testing the efficacy of tamoxifen (20 mg/day) with or without 4-HPR (200 or 400 mg/day).
The availability of different agents that are potentially independently capable of inhibiting tumour occurrence and/or progression in hormone-dependent and independent breast cancers raises new clinical challenges. The hypothesis that tamoxifen could prevent ER-

positive tumours and retinoids ER-negative ones is at present purely theoretical but preclinical data suggest that the combination is worthy of further investigation.

Retinoids in Breast Cancer Therapy

Some of the preclinical data that justified the use of retinoids in breast cancer chemoprevention also led to the use of retinoids alone or in combination with tamoxifen in patients with breast carcinoma. In addition, retinoids have been shown both to induce the synthesis of TGF-beta, a negative growth factor for breast cancer cells [75], and to inhibit IGF-1-induced growth in the breast cancer cell line MCF-7 [76]. Phase II trials of 13-*cis* RA and 4-HPR used as single agents in patients with advanced breast carcinoma were negative [31, 77]. However, in a subset of patients studied in the trials using 4-HPR in stage I breast cancer discussed above it was demonstrated by Torrisi et al. [78] that therapy with 4-HPR significantly lowered circulating IGF-1. Tamoxifen has also been demonstrated to decrease the levels of this factor in the same patient population [79]. On the basis of these findings as well as preclinical observations of increased activity of retinoid/tamoxifen combinations in breast carcinoma [68], clinical trials to explore this combination have been initiated. Cobleigh et al. recently published the initial results of a phase I trial of 4-HPR and tamoxifen [80]. No maximally tolerated dose was obtained in this trial, and additional trials to establish the toxicity of this combination at maximally tolerated doses as well as its biological and clinical effects are under way.

Bladder Cancer

Retinoids in the Prevention of Bladder Carcinoma

Numerous studies have suggested correlations between the development of invasive bladder cancer and low serum values of retinol, retinol-binding protein, and carotenoid [81].

The effect of retinoids on urinary bladder tumours has been demonstrated in several animal model systems [82,83] and has been investigated in clinical studies [8,84]. The results of published studies suggest a moderate activity of retinoids in preventing recurrence of superficial bladder cancer (in most cases the retinoid used was etretinate), although the benefits are probably overshadowed by the considerable toxicity which resulted in the use of suboptimal doses. A few pilot studies have investigated the activity of retinol or retinoic acid in the treatment of non-resected superficial bladder cancer, with complete remissions being reported [8]. In one trial isotretinoin (0.5 mg/kg/day) was used as a prophylactic agent in patients with recurrent low-grade lesions. Unfortunately, after 22 patients had been studied, this trial was prematurely discontinued due to apparent cutaneous and ophthalmological (blepharoconjunctivitis) side-effects [85].

Three small randomised trials investigated the use of etretinate (50 mg day) in the prophylaxis of recurrent superficial bladder cancer. In the first study, 17 of 47 patients had to stop drug intake due to toxicity [86]. It was not possible to demonstrate any difference in the recurrence rate in this small group of patients. Also in the second study the initial daily dose of 50 mg was reduced to 25 mg due to side-effects occurring during the first month of therapy [87]. The investigators concluded that compared to the baseline values established for the 2 years preceding the trial, etretinate produced a reduction in the number of tumours at cystoscopy. A third randomised, double-blind trial was conducted on 86 patients [88]. Dose reductions to 25 mg were required in 90% of patients. There were fewer multiple tumour recurrences in the etretinate group: 17% versus 48% ($p < 0.02$). A larger randomised study on 270 patients comparing etretinate at a daily dose of 20 mg for 3 years versus no treatment was conducted in Italy [89]. Preliminary results show a significant reduction of recurrences in the retinoid arm (49 versus 80, $p < 0.004$). Toxicity was common but never severe.

In summary, low-dose etretinate therapy may have moderate activity in the prophylaxis of superficial bladder cancer. The results may be promising if the low dose (25 mg daily) employed is considered. Recently, particular attention has been focused on the synthetic retinoid 4-hydroxy-phenyl retinamide (4-HPR). *In vitro* experiments show that 4-HPR can significantly inhibit the proliferation of human bladder cancer cells [90]. Fenretinide can reach high concentrations in the rodent bladder [91] and proves to be one of the most potent and safe retinamides against bladder carcinogenesis in the mouse [92]. The clinical activity of 4-HPR in superficial bladder cancer has recently been investigated in a phase IIa trial using DNA flow cytometry as an intermediate endpoint [93]. A significant reduction in the hyperdiploid fraction of bladder washed cells was observed in patients treated with 4-HPR. A randomised trial using DNA-flow cytometry as a surrogate endpoint is ongoing.

Retinoids in the Therapy of Bladder Carcinoma

There is only a limited amount of information regarding retinoid biology in bladder cancer, and very little clinical experience with therapy of bladder cancer using retinoids. RAR expression was documented in more than one half of bladder tumours examined [94]. Objective responses in patients with recurrent bladder cancer have been achieved with etretinate therapy [95].

Based on synergistic antitumour effects *in vitro* of the combination of fluorouracil and IFN-alpha with either 13-*cis* RA or 4-HPR, a phase I trial of the combination (using 13-*cis* RA) has been conducted [96] in preparation of comparative clinical trials designed to evaluate any particular contribution by the addition of retinoids to the cytotoxic agent regimen. Escalating doses of oral 13-*cis* RA were combined with the combination chemo- and biological therapy; significant toxicity required dose reductions in a majority of the patients.

Other Malignancies

Potential for Retinoids in Prostate Carcinoma Chemoprevention and Therapy

It has long been known that retinoids are capable of reversing carcinogen-induced morphological changes in prostate cells [97]. In addition, in a chemoprevention study 4-HPR decreased the incidence of primary prostate carcinoma from 88% to 21% in carcinogen-treated animals [98]. Again, based on the demonstrated inhibitory effects of retinoids on prostate cancer cell line growth as well as the induction of differentiation of some of these same cell lines, phase II clinical trials of RA for treatment of prostate cancer have been initiated.

Retinoids in the Therapy of Germ Cell Tumours

Based on extensive preclinical information that human embryonal carcinoma cell lines can be induced to differentiate by retinoids, clinical trials of retinoids in patients with chemotherapy-refractory germ cell tumours have been conducted. 13-*cis* RA therapy resulted in no objective responses in 15 patients with advanced germ cell tumours, although 4 patients experienced prolonged disease stabilisation for periods of 5 to 7.5 months [99].

Retinoids in the Therapy of Primary Central Nervous System Malignancies

Some cell lines derived from cultured human gliomas show growth inhibition in response to RA; one author has suggested that a possible mechanism may be related to the retinoid-associated modulation of the phosphotyrosine kinase activity of the epidermal growth factor receptor [100]. The combination of interferon beta with RA has been shown by these same investigators to be synergistic against cultured glioma cell lines *in vitro* [100]. Interferon beta as a single agent has produced objective responses in patients with advanced gliomas, while interferon alpha has been essentially inactive when studied in the same situation [101]. In a recent clinical trial conducted by Levin et al., objective responses were noted with 13-*cis* RA administered as a single agent [102]. As a result, a clinical trial of the combination of interferon-beta and 13-*cis* RA has been initiated.

Retinoids in the Therapy of Sarcomas

The antiangiogenic properties of retinoids have led to the study of RA in patients with AIDS-associated Kaposi's sarcoma. Oral 13-*cis* RA had no activity in 6 patients with this malignancy [103]. However, topical RA (1% gel) produced more than 50% reductions in the size of cutaneous lesions in 7 of 8 patients with epidemic Kaposi's sarcoma [104]. Based on these observations, phase II studies of RA alone and in combination with interferon alpha in patients with AIDS-associated KS are under way.

Retinoids in the Therapy of Neuroblastoma

In one report, 3 patients with bone marrow involvement by neuroblastoma showed 1 to 3 log decreases in bone marrow involvement following 13-*cis* RA treatment at a dose of 100 mg/m^2 [105,106]. To date no responses have been reported in patients with advanced disease. One patient with neuroblastoma initiated on therapy in early relapse remained free of detectable disease for 2 years while receiving 13-*cis* RA. Clinical trials of 13-*cis* RA in neuroblastoma are currently under way both in the United States and in Europe. In an ongoing Children's Cancer Group clinical trial, patients with advanced neuroblastoma are randomised to receive either no additional therapy or 13-*cis* RA (125 mg/m^2/d for 2 weeks with 2 weeks of rest) for 24 weeks following completion of intensive cytotoxic therapy. The European Neuroblastoma Study Group is conducting a randomised trial comparing 13-*cis* RA (0.75 mg/kg/day) as daily maintenance for 2 years with a placebo in patients who have achieved either complete response or a good partial response following cytotoxic therapy.

A Perspective: Retinoids in Chemoprevention and Therapy

In the future of cancer research, chemoprevention and biological therapy of solid tumours will hopefully share a greater amount of energy and financial resources. The continuous progress of molecular biology and cytogenetics has provided clinicians with extremely powerful techniques to identify individuals at risk, detect precancerous or non-invasive lesions in the target field, and monitor the results of intervention.

A number of cytogenetic and molecular biology studies have demonstrated that specific and consistent genetic changes may be identified in the various steps of epithelial carcinogenesis. Based on this finding, there is now the chance to design a new generation of clinical trials using genetic biomarkers to identify optimal candidates for specific chemoprevention programmes, and also to monitor the results of intervention in the short and intermediate term.

A panel of new preventive agents are ready to be tested in optimal combination schedules, with the aim of counteracting each of the different types and stages of carcinogenesis. From this point of view, it appears justified to incorporate chemopreventive agents in randomised trials testing new adjuvant strategies as well as multimodality treatments.

Combination of retinoids with other substances characterised by different mechanisms of action, such as cytokines, antioxidants, vitamin D analogues and hormones, represents a most promising field of clinical investigation.

REFERENCES

1 Hong WK, Bromer RH, Amato DA: Paterns of relapse in locally advanced head and neck cancer patients who achieved complete remission after combined modality therapy. Cancer 1985 (56): 1242-1245

2 De Vries N: The magnitude of the problem. In: de Vries N and Glukman JL (eds) Multiple Primary Tumors in the Head and Neck. Thieme, Stuttgart 1990 pp 1-29

3 Slaughter DP, Southwick HW, Smejkal W: "Field cancerization" in oral stratified squamous epithelium: clinical implications of multicentric origin. Cancer 1953 (6):963-968

4 De Vries N, Snow GB: Multiple primary tumors in laryngeal cancer. J Laryngol Otol 1986 (100):915-917

5 McDonald S, Haie C, Rubin P, Nelson D, Divers LD: Second malignant tumors in patients with laryngeal carcinoma: diagnosis, treatment and prevention. Int J Radiat Oncol Biol Phys 1989 (17):457-465

6 Pairolero P, Williams DE, Bergstrahl EJ et al: Post-surgical stage I bronchogenic carcinoma: morbid implications of recurrent disease. Ann Thorac Surg 1984 (38):331-338

7 Bertram JS, Kolonel LN, Meyskens FL: Rationale and strategies for chemoprevention of cancer in humans. Cancer Res 1987 (47):3012-3031

8 Lippman SM, Kessler JF, Meyskens FL: Retinoids as preventive and therapeutic anticancer agents (part II). Cancer Treat Rep 1987 (71):493-515

9 Sundaresan V, Ganly P, Hasleton P et al: p53 and chromosome 3 abnormalities, characteristic of malignant lung tumours, are detectable in preinvasive lesions of the bronchus. Oncogene 1992 (7): 1989-1997

10 Sozzi G, Miozzo M, Donghi R et al: Deletions of 17p and p53 mutations in preneoplastic lesions of the lung. Cancer Res 1992 (52):6079-6082

11 Pastorino U, Sozzi G, Miozzo M et al: Genetic changes in lung cancer. J Cell Biochem 1993 (17F): 237-248

12 Chung KY, Mukhopadhyay T, Kim J et al: Discordant p53 gene mutations in primary head and neck cancers and corresponding second primary cancers of the upper aerodigestive tract. Can Res 1993 (53):1676-1683

13 Lee JS, Lippman SM, Hong WK et al: Determination of biomarkers for intermediate end points in chemoprevention trials. Cancer Res 1992 (52 suppl 9): 2707s-2710s

14 Moriarity M, Dunn J, Derregh A, Lambe R, Brick I: Etretinate in treatment of actinic keratoses: a double-blind cross over study. Lancet 1982 (1): 364-365

15 Watson AB: Preventive effect of etretinate therapy on multiple actinic keratoses. Cancer Detect Prev 1986 (9):161-165

16 Kraemer KH, Di Giovanna JJ, Moshell AN, Tarone RE, Peck GL: Prevention of skin cancer in xeroderma pigmentosum with the use of oral isotretinoin. N Engl J Med 1988 (318):1633-1637

17 Tangrea JA, Edwards BK, Taylor PR et al: Long-term therapy with low-dose isotretinoin for prevention of basal cell carcinoma: a multicenter clinical trial. Isotretinoin-Basal Cell Carcinoma Study Group. JNCI 1992 (84):328-332

18 Nava M, Fabrizio T, Arioli N et al: Chemoprevention of basal cell carcinoma by prolonged administration of the synthetic retinoid fenretinide (4-HPR). In: De Palo G, Sporn M, Veronesi U (eds) Progress and Perspectives in Chemoprevention of Cancer. Serono Symposia Publications from Raven Press, Vol 79, New York 1992, pp 161-170

19 Peck R and Bollag W: Potentiation of retinoid-induced differentiation of H2-60 and U937 cell lines by cytokines. Eur J Cancer 1991 (27):53-57

20 Lippman SM, Parkinson DR, Itri LM et al: 13-cis-Retinoic acid and interferon alpha-2a: Effective combination therapy for advanced squamous cell carcinoma of the skin. JNCI 1992 (84):235-241

21 Lippman SM and DiGiovanna JJ: Retinoids in skin cancer. In: Hong WK and Lotan R (eds) Retinoids in Oncology. Marcel Dekker Inc, New York 1993 pp 179-202

22 Toma S, Palumbo R, Vincenti M et al: Efficacy of recombinant alpha-interferon 2a and 13-cis-retinoic acid in the treatment of squamous cell carcinoma. Ann Oncol 1994 (in press)

23 Sankowski A, Janik P, Jeziorska M et al: The results of topical application of 13-cis-retinoic acid on basal cell carcinoma. A correlation of the clinical effect with histopathological examination and serum retinol level. Neoplasma 1987 (34):485-489

24 Peck G, DiGiovanna J, Sarnoff D et al: Treatment and prevention of basal cell carcinoma with oral isotretinoin. J Am Acad Dermatol 1988 (19):176-185

25 Hodak E, Ginzburg A, David M et al: Etretinate treatment of the nevoid basal cell carcinoma syndrome. Int J Dermatol 1987 (26):606-609

26 Felix E, Cohen M, Loyd B: Inhibition of the growth and development of a transplantable murine melanoma by vitamin A. Science 1975 (189):886-887

27 Meyskens F and Fuller B: Characterization of the effects of different retinoids on the growth and differentiation of a human melanoma cell line and selected subclones. Cancer Res 1980 (40):2194-2196

28 Wang Z,Cao Y, D'Urso CM, Ferrone S: Differential susceptibility of cultured human melanoma cell lines to enhancement by retinoic acid of intercellular adhesion molecule 1 expression. Cancer Res 1992 (52):4766-4772

29 Levine N, Meyskens F: Topical vitamin-A-acid therapy for cutaneous metastatic melanoma. Lancet 1980 (2):224-226

30 Goodman G: Phase II trial of retinol in patients with advanced cancer. Cancer Treat Rep 1986 (70): 1023-1024

31 Modiano M, Dalton W, Lippman S et al: Phase II study of fenretinide (n-[4-hydroxyphenyl] retinamide) in advanced breast cancer and melanoma. Invest New Drugs 1990 (8):317-319

32 Meyskens F, Kopecky K, Costanzi J et al: A randomized phase III trial of high dose vitamin A vesus placebo for stage I malignant melanoma. Proc Am Soc Clin Oncol 1988 (7):247 (abstract)

33 Dhingra K, Papadopoulos N, Lippman S, Lotan R, Legha SS: Phase II study of alpha-interferon and 13-cis-retinoic acid in metastatic melanoma. Invest New Drugs 1993 (11): 39-43
34 Hong WK, Endicott J, Itri L et al: 13-cis-retinoic acid in the treatment of oral leukoplakia. New Engl J Med 1986 (315):1501-1505
35 Lippman SM, Batsakis JG, Toth BB et al: Comparison of low-dose isotretinoin with beta carotene to prevent oral carcinogenesis. N Engl J Med 1993 (328):15-20
36 Chiesa F, Tradati N, Marazza M et al: Prevention of local relapses and new localisations of oral leukoplakia with the synthetic retinoid fenretinide (4-HPR). Preliminary results. Oral Oncology - Eur J Cancer 1992 (28B):97-102
37 Hong W, Lippman S, Itri L et al: Prevention of secondary primary tumor with isotretinoin in squamous-cell carcinoma of the head and neck. N Engl J Med 1990 (323):795-801
38 Benner SE, Lee JS, Goepfert H, Hong WK: Long term follow up: 13-cis-retinoic acid (cRA) prevention of second primary tumors (SPT) following squamous cell carcinoma of the head and neck (SCCHN). Proc ASCO 1993 (12):900
39 Bolla M, Lefur R, Van Ton J et al: Prevention of second primary with etretinate in squamous cell carcinoma of oral cavity and oropharynx. A randomized double blind study. Proc Second International Cancer Chemo-Prevention Conference (CCPC-93). Berlin, April 28-30, 1993 p76
40 Sacks P, Oke V, Calkins D et al: Effects of beta-all-trans retinoic acid on growth, proliferation and cell death in a multicellular tumor spheroid model for squamous carcinomas. J Cell Physiol 1990 (144):237-243
41 Meyskens FL, Gilmartin E, Alberts DS: Activity of isootretinoin against squamous cell cancers and preneoplastic lesions. Cancer Treat Rep 66:1315-1319, 1982
42 Lippman S, Kessler J, Meyskens J: Retinoids as preventive and therapeutic anticancer agents. Cancer Treat Rep 1987 (71):391-405
43 Lippman S and Meyskens F: Treatment of advanced squamous cell carcinoma of the skin with isotretinoin. Ann Intern Med 1987 (107):499-502
44 Komiyama S, Hiroto I, Ryu S et al: Synergistic combination therapy of 5-fluorouracil, vitamin A, and cobalt-60 radiation for head and neck tumors. Auris Nasus Larynx 1985 (12):5239-5243
45 Thatcher N, Blackledge G, Crowther D: Advanced recurrent squamous cell carcinoma of the head and neck. Results of a chemotherapeutic regimen with adriamycin, bleomycin, 5-fluorouracil, methotrexate, and vitamin A. Cancer 1980 (46):1324-1328
46 Mills E: The modifying efffect of beta-carotene on radiation and chemotherapy-induced oral mucositis. Br J Cancer 1988 (57):416-417
47 Voravud V, Lippman SM, Wever R et al: Phase I trial of 13-cis-retinoic acid plus interferon-alpha in recurrent head and neck cancer. Invest New Drugs 1993 (11):57-60
48 Greenwald P, Sondik E, Lynch BS: Diet and chemoprevention in NCI's research strategy to achieve national cancer control objectives. Ann Rev Public Health 1986 (7):267-291
49 Arnold AM, Browman GP, Levine MN et al: The efect of the synthetic retinoid etretinate on sputum cytology: results from a randomised trial. Br J Cancer 1992 (65):737-743
50 Lee JS, Benner SE, Lippman SM et al: A randomised placebo-controlled chemoprevention trial of 13-cis-retinoic acid (cRA) in bronchial squamous metaplasia. Proc ASCO 1993 (13):1117
51 Pastorino U, Infante I, Maioli M et al: Adjuvant treatment of stage I lung cancer with high dose vitamin A JCO 1993 (11):1216-1222
52 De Vries N, Van Zandwijk N, Pastorino U: The EUROSCAN Study. Br J Cancer 1991 (64):985-989
53 Lippman SM, Benner SE, Hong WK: Chemoprevention strategies in lung carcinogenesis. Chest 1993 (103):15S-19S
54 Munker M, Munker R, Saxton R et al: Effect of recombinant monokines, lymphokines and other agents on clonal proliferation of human lung cancer cell lines. Cancer Res 1987 (47):4081-4085
55 Micksche M, Cerni, Kokron O. Stimulation of immune response in lung cancer patients by vitamin A therapy. Oncology 1977 (34):234-238
56 Grunberg S, Itri L: Phase II study of isotretinoin in the treatent of advanced nonsmall cell lung cancer. Cancer Treat Rep 1987 (71):1097-1098
57 Doyle L, Giangiulo D, Hussain A et al: Differentiation of human variant small cell cancer cell lines to a classic morphology by retinoic acid. Cancer Res 1989 (49):6745-6751
58 Lippman SM, Kavanagh JJ, Paredes-Espinoza et al: 13-cis-Retinoic acid plus interferon alpha-2a: highly active systemic therapy for squamous cell carcinoma of the cervix. JNCI 1992 (84):241-245
59 Kavanagh JJ, Kudelka AP, Lippman SM, Krakoff IH: Retinoids and cervical cancer. In: Hong WK and Lotan R (eds) Retinoids in Oncology. Marcel Dekker Inc, New York 1993 pp 271-278
60 LaCroix A, Lippman M: Binding of retinoids to human breast cancer cell lines and their effects on cell growth. J Clin Invest 1980 (65):586-591
61 Marth C, Bock G, Daxenbichler G: Effect of 4-hydroxyphenylretinamide and retinoic acid on proliferation and cell cycle of cultured human breast cancer cells JNCI 1985 (75):871-875
62 Fontana J, Miranda D, Mezu A: Retinoic acid inhibition of human breast carcinoma proliferation is accompanied by inhibition of the synthesis of a Mr 39,000 protein. Cancer Res 1990 (50):1977-1982
63 LaCroix A, Doskas C, Bhat P: Inhibition of growth of established N-methyl-N-nitrosourea-induced mammary cancer in rats by retinoic acid and ovariectomy. Cancer Res 1990 (50):5731-5734
64 Halter S, Fraker L, Adcock D et al: Effect of retinoids on xenotransplanted human mammary carcinoma cells in athymic mice. Cancer Res 1988 (48):3733-3736
65 Costa A: Biological approaches to breast cancer prevention. The Breast 1992 (1):119-123
66 Sporn MB and Newton DL: Chemoprevention of cancer with retinoids. Fed Proc 1979 (38):2528-2534

67 Moon RC, Thompson HJ, Becci PL et al: N-(4-hydroxyphenyl) retinamide, a new retinoid for prevention of breast cancer. Cancer Res 1979 (39):1339-1346
68 Ratko TA, Detrisac CJ, Dinger NM et al: Chemopreventive efficacy of combined retinoid and tamoxifen treatment following surgical excision of a primary mammary cancer in female rats. Cancer Res 1989 (49):4472-4476
69 Costa A: Retinoids and breast cancer. In: Hong WK and Lotan R (eds) Retinoids in Oncology. Marcel Dekker Inc, New York 1993 pp 299-322
70 Formelli F, Carsana R, Costa A et al: Plasma retinol level reduction by the synthetic retinoid fenretinide: a one year follow-up study of breast cancer patients. Cancer Res 1989 (48):6149-6152
71 Berni R and Formelli F: In vitro interaction of fenretinide with plasma retinolbinding protein and its functional consequences. FEBS 1992 (308):43-45
72 Veronesi U, De Palo G, Costa A et al: Chemoprevention of breast cancer with retinoids. JNCI Monograph 1992 (12):93-97
73 Fisher B, Costantino J, Redmond C et al: A randomized clinical trial evaluating tamoxifen in the treatment of patients with node-negative breast cancer who have estrogen-receptor-positive tumours. New Engl J Med 1989 (320):479-484
74 Early Breast Cancer Trialists' Collaborative Group: Systemic treatment of early breast cancer by hormonal, cytotoxic, or immune therapy: 133 randomised trials involving 31,000 recurrences and 24,000 deaths among 75,000 women. Lancet 1992 (339):1-15
75 Knabbe C, Lippman ME, Wakefield LM et al: Evidence that TGF-beta is a hormonally regulated negative growth-factor in human breast cancer cells. Cell 1987 (48):417-428
76 Adamo ML, Shao Z-M, Lanau F et al: Insulin-like growth factor-1 (IGF-1) and retinoic acid modulation of IGF-binding protiens (IGFBPs): IFGBP-2,-3, and -4 gene expression and protein secretion in a breast cancer cell line. Endocrinology 1992 (131):1858-1866
77 Cassidy J, Lippman M, LaCroix A et al: Phase II trial of 13-cis-retinoid acid in metastatic breast cancer. Eur J Cancer Clin Oncol 1092 (18):925-928
78 Torrisi R, Pensa F, Orengo MA et al: The synthetic retinoid fenretinide lowers plasma insulin-like growth factor I levels in breast cancer patients. Cancer Res 1993 (53):4769-4771
79 Pollak M, Costantino J, Polychronakos C et al: Effect of tamoxifen on serum insulin-like growth factor I levels in stage I breast cancer patients. JNCI 1990 (82):1693-1697
80 Cobleigh MA, Dowlatshahi K, Deutsch TA et al: Phase I/II trial of tamoxifen with or without fenretinide, an analog of vitamin A, in women with metastatic breast cancer. J Clin Oncol 1993 (11): 474-477
81 Tyler H, Notley R, Schweitzer F et al: Vitamin A status and bladder cancer. Eur J Surg Oncol 1986 (12):35-41
82 Moon RC, McCormick DL, Metha RG: Inhibition of carcinogenesis by retinoids. Cancer Res 1983 (43 suppl 5):2469-2475
83 Hicks RM: The scientific basis for regarding vitamin A and its analogues as anticarcinogenic agents. Proc Nutr Soc 1983 (42):83-93
84 Malone WF, Kelloff GJ, Pierson H et al: Chemoprevention of bladder cancer. Cancer 1987 (60):650-657
85 Prout GR Jr and Barton BA: 13-cis-Retinoic acid in chemoprevention of superficial bladder cancer. J Cell Biochem 1992 (16 suppl I):148-152
86 Pedersen H, Wolf H, Jensen SK et al: Administration of a retinoid as prophylaxis of recurrent non-invasive bladder tumors. Scand J Urol Nephr 1984 (18):121-123
87 Alfthan O, Tarkkanen J, Grohn P et al: Tigason (etretinate) in prevention of recurrence of superficial bladder tumors. A double-blind clinical trial. Eur Urol 1983 (9):6
88 Studer UE, Biedermann C, Chollet D et al: Prevention of recurrent superficial bladder tumors by oral etretinate: preliminary results of a randomized, double-blind multicenter study in Switzerland. J Urol 1983 (131):47-49
89 Di Silverio F, von Heland M, La Pera G et al: Retinoids and prophylaxis of superficial bladder tumor recurrence. In: Boccardo F, Giuliani L, Pescatore D, Santi L (eds) New Trends in Diagnosis and Treatment of Bladder Cancer. Sympomed Verlag, Munchen 1994 (in press)
90 McCormick AM, Patel M et al: Metabolism of 4-hydroxyphenyl-retinamide and retinoic acid in vivo and in cultured bladder carcinoma cells. Fed Proc 1985 (44):1672
91 Hultin TA, May CM, Moon RC: N-(4-hydroxyphenyl)-all-trans-retinamide pharmacokinetics in female rats and mice. Drug Metab Dispos Biol Fate Chem 1986 (14):714-717
92 Moon RC, McCormick DL, Becci PJ et al: Influence of 15 retinoic acid amides on urinary bladder carcinogenesis. Carcinogenesis 1982 (3):1469-1472
93 Decensi A, Bruno S, Costantini M et al: Phase IIa study of fenretinide in superficial bladder cancer, using DNA flow cytometry as an intermediate end point. JNCI 1994 (86):138-140
94 Fagg S, Hughes A, Fielding J et al: Retinoic acid receptor in human bladder tumors. Clin Oncol 1982 (8):329-334
95 Schaerer R, Swiercz P, Mousseau M et al: Is acid aromatic vitamin A (etretinate) active in low grade malignant bladder carcinoma. Cancer Chemother Pharmacol 1982 (9):50 (abstract)
96 Recondo G, Logothetis C, Hossan E et al: Results of the phase I trial combining 13-cis-retinoic acid (13-cRA) with 5-fluorouracil (5-FU), alpha-inerferon 2b (Intron) in patients with chemotherapy refractory transitional cell carcinoma of the bladder. Proc Am Soc Clin Oncol 1991 (10):174 (abstract)
97 Lasnitzki I: The influence of a hypervitaminosis on the effect of 20-methyl-cholanthrene on mouse prostate glands grown in vitro. Br J Cancer 1955 (9):434-441
98 Pollard M, Luckert P, Sporn M: Prevention of

primary prostate cancer in Lobund-Wistar rats by N-(4-hydroxyphenyl)retinamide. Cancer Res 1991 (51):3610-3611
99 Gold E, Bosl G, Itri L: Phase II trial of 13-cis-retinoic acid in patients with advanced nonseminomatous germ cell tumors. Cancer Treat Rep 1984 (68):1287-1288
100 Yung W, Lotan R, Lee P et al: Modulation of growth and epidermal growth factor receptor activity by retinoic acid in human glioma cells. Cancer Res 1989 (49):1014-1019
101 Yung WK, Prados M, Levin VA et al: Intravenous recombinant interferon beta in patients with recurrent malignant gliomas: a phase I/II study. J Clin Oncol 1991 (9):1945-1949
102 Yung WK, Simaga N, Levin VA: 13-cis-retinoic acid: A new potentially effective agent for recurrent malignant astrocytomas. Proc ASCO 1993 (12): 497 (abstract)
103 Biegler J, Volverding P, Itri L: Failure of isotretinoin in Kaposi's sarcoma. Lancet 1984 (2):641
104 Bonhomme L, Fredj G, Averous S et al: Topical treatment of epidemic Kaposi's sarcoma with all-trans-retinoic acid. Ann Oncol 1991 (2):234-235
105 Reynolds C, Kane D, Einhorn P et al: Response of neuroblastoma to retinoic acid in vitro and in vivo. In: Evans A, D'Angio G, Knudson A et al (eds) Advances in Neuroblastoma Research, Vol 3. A Liss, New York 1991 pp 203-211
106 Reynolds C, Matthay K, Crouse V et al: Response of neuroblastoma bone marrow metastases to 13-cis-retinoic acid. Proc Am Soc Clin Oncol 1990 (9):54 (abstract)

Retinoids in Oncology: Conclusions and Future Directions

Laurent Degos [1] and David R. Parkinson [2]

1 Institut Universitaire d'Hématologie, Hôpital St. Louis, 1, Avenue Claude Vellefaux, 75010 Paris, France
2 Investigational Drug Branch, Division of Cancer Treatment, National Cancer Institute, Bethesda, MD 20892, U.S.A.

Cancer is overall the net result of disturbances in normal processes of cellular growth and differentiation, processes in which natural retinoids play a major homeostatic role. The authors of this monograph have provided an overview of the current understanding of retinoid biology with particular reference to the use of this class of agents in the prevention and treatment of malignancy. It is clear from the discussions in this book that, although there have been dramatic increases both in our understanding of these agents and in our experience with their use in therapeutics, much remains to be learned. As discussed by Arthur Zelent, many of the molecular components of the retinoid signalling pathways have been identified. Still to be defined, however, is the extent of the interactions between retinoid and other nuclear receptors, and the nature and importance of differences in expression of different retinoid receptors in different tissues. The complexities of this system will continue to present challenges in predicting the net biological effects of particular therapeutic interventions in the clinical setting. The recent demonstrations of the negative regulation by all-*trans* retinoic acid of AP-1-responsive genes, the role of retinoid nuclear receptor phosphorylation in receptor activation, and interactions between retinoid receptors and other nuclear receptors, including proto-oncogenes such as v-*erb*A, are probably only the beginning of increased appreciation of the linkage between retinoid signalling pathways and other critical cellular pathways involved in growth and differentiation. A further complexity relates to the possibility that retinoid-mediated effects can be induced through mechanisms other than the retinoid receptors, for example through direct retinoylation of intracellular proteins. Understanding of retinoid biology continues to increase at a remarkable rate, and it is clear that this improved basic understanding of the biology of this class of agents will continue to affect our estimation of their potential uses and limitations in cancer therapy.

As reviewed by Reuben Lotan, the powerful effects of retinoids *in vitro* suggest that they could be useful in the restoration of malignant cells to patterns of normal growth and differentiation when used either alone or in combination with other agents active in regulation of these cellular processes. Translating these preclinical findings into positive clinical effects with respect to cancer prevention or treatment has continued to present formidable challenges. Some dramatic successes have emerged already, the most dramatic, of course, is the remarkable clinical benefit achieved with the use of all-*trans* retinoic acid in the therapy of acute promyelocytic leukaemia, as discussed by de Thé and colleagues in this monograph. However, the limitations of this therapeutic approach have also rapidly become evident. Recognition and development of appropriate therapy for the "retinoic acid syndrome" has decreased the incidence of one source of morbidity and mortality. However, in the initial clinical experience, the incidence of early death in patients presenting with APL has not been decreased with all-*trans* RA as compared to that observed with classic cytotoxic chemotherapeutic approaches. Beyond the risk of the "retinoic acid syndrome", patients remain at great risk for bleeding in the first hours or days after presenting with this leukaemia, and the effects of all-*trans* RA may not be rapid enough to completely eliminate this problem. Although the prolonged period of risk from infection and bleeding may be less with all-*trans* RA used alone, it rapidly became clear that induction of remission with all-*trans* RA alone resulted in many patients in remissions of only a few months' duration. The reasons why patients fail have only been partially defined. Based on the demonstrated stable pharmacokinetics of 13-*cis* retinoic acid over time, it was a great surprise when the Memorial Sloan-Kettering investigators first demonstrated the rapid induction of metabolism of all-*trans* RA. Since that first demonstration, much has been learned about the particular pharmacokinetics of this agent, and as discussed in the chapter by Pastorino et al. a number of strategies, including concomitant use of P450 inhibitors and intermittent dosing schedules, have been developed in an attempt to overcome this apparent pharmacological problem. This phenomenon certainly brings into question the value of long-term maintenance therapy with all-*trans* RA, although it is curious that some patients with demonstrated dramatic falls in their all-*trans* RA levels over time continue to experience retinoid side-effects, suggesting continued retinoid biological activity. However, it seems clear that besides the pharmacological problems, a central problem in patient relapse must also relate to biological resistance, and this phenomenon is worthy of much further study than it has attracted to date. It is possible that studies with newer retinoids due to enter clinical trial, including 9-*cis* retinoic acid, will provide evidence for important clinical activity without the pharmacological and biological disadvantages of all-*trans* RA.

It seems also clear from the early Chinese, French and American data, that an important priority for continued therapeutic development in patients with APL is the study of the combined use of all-*trans* RA and cytotoxic chemotherapy. The randomised French studies described in the chapter by de Thé et al. represent the best evidence accumulated to date for the advantages of this combined strategy; important evidence in this regard will also be forthcoming from the large Intergroup study which is currently ongoing. Finally, as discussed in this monograph, the mechanism of the beneficial effect of all-*trans* RA in APL is still not defined and must remain an important research goal, since, although at this point APL appears to be a unique situation, the biological lessons to be learned may be more widely relevant.

Another important lead to the use of retinoids in cancer therapy has come from the observations of the investigators from Houston and Guadalajara concerning the effect of the combination of interferon alpha and 13-*cis* RA on squamous cell carcinoma of the cervix. Many issues remain to be resolved with this strategy as well; these include clinical questions regarding the generalisability of these observations to the cervical carcinoma observed in North American and European populations, the effect of prior chemotherapy or radiation therapy on the activity of these agents, the durability of the responses, and the best way to integrate this approach into more conventional approaches to this malignancy. In addition, extension of these observations to other squamous cell malignancies with similar epidemiological backgrounds, such as penile and vulvar cancers, will be important in future studies. While the initial information regarding squamous cell malignancies other than those of the skin and cervix is limited, the first reports are not encouraging. For this reason, it becomes particularly important to define the biological basis of the activity of these agents in cervical and dermatological malignancies.

Understanding of these mechanisms, as with the operative mechanism of response to all-*trans* RA in APL, is critical to the development of new retinoids and related molecules for cancer therapy and prevention. Without a biological target for therapeutic development, clinical development will remain largely empirical and very inefficient.

A large number of phase II trials of all-*trans* RA and other retinoids used alone or in combination are currently under way in a range of solid tumours and haematological malignancies; the majority of these trials include laboratory investigations in addition to the more conventional clinical response endpoints. It is hoped that these trials will cumulatively provide significant information on the activity of these agents in patients with advanced disease, and on their biological effects on the various tumours.

Considerable efforts are currently being expended to the development of retinoids specific for individual RAR or RXR receptors, or for each class of receptors. Whether these specific agonists (or the complementary antagonists) will prove of greater therapeutic benefit in humans with malignancy remains problematic at this point; however, they will clearly be important tools in the dissection of the biology of this class of agents. The recent introduction into clinical trial of vitamin D3 analogues which apparently retain many of the differentiation-related effects without the severe hypercalcaemia inducing effects of this hormone will open additional possibilities for combination therapy if indicated by preclinical studies. Finally, the major retinoid-based chemoprevention trials which are currently under way should provide important new information on the successes and limitations of the currently used agents for prevention. As with therapy, the greatest advances will no doubt be led by increased understanding of the true nature of the biological effects of this class of agents in the premalignant and malignant setting.

MIX
Papier aus verantwortungsvollen Quellen
Paper from responsible sources
FSC® C105338

If you have any concerns about our products,
you can contact us on
ProductSafety@springernature.com

In case Publisher is established outside the EU,
the EU authorized representative is:
Springer Nature Customer Service Center GmbH
Europaplatz 3, 69115 Heidelberg, Germany

Printed by Libri Plureos GmbH
in Hamburg, Germany